Breastfeeding for Public Heal

Health visitors play a crucial role in supporting mothers who choose to breastfeed and their families. This accessible text enables readers to practise confidently in this vital area, focusing on underpinning knowledge and parent-centred counselling skills, and understanding cultural contexts.

Breastfeeding a child improves the lifelong health of a population, and promoting breastfeeding is an important area of public health practice. *Breastfeeding for Public Health* incorporates the voices of health visitors, mothers and fathers to give insight into common practical challenges faced and suggestions for overcoming or working around them. Presenting up-to-date research, it explores the practical skills needed by health visitors to support mothers with breastfeeding; how to develop the communication skills and self-awareness necessary to build successful and trusting relationships with women and their families; why breastfeeding is so important for babies' and mothers' health and psychological attachment, closeness and long-term mental health; what we know about the content of breastmilk and the positive effect it has on the baby's gut microbiome, which in turn benefits the infant's long-term health and helps to protect against non-communicable diseases; the role of the father and grandparents in successfully initiating and sustaining breastfeeding; and how cultural awareness and sensitivity can influence practice for the better.

Written by an experienced volunteer and practitioner with decades of experience as a health visitor and breastfeeding counsellor, this text is ideal for students taking Specialist Community and Public Health Nursing courses. It is also an important reference for practising health visitors.

Alison Spiro has worked as a health visitor and an NCT breastfeeding counsellor, recently acting as a specialist health visitor and infant feeding lead in two NHS trusts, taking them both to become Baby Friendly accredited by UNICEF. She did a doctorate in social anthropology and studied breastfeeding in Indian families in London and India. Recognised as a Queen's Nurse in 2014, she is now a professional advisor for Best Beginnings and the Institute of Health Visiting, and a volunteer in breastfeeding support groups and training peer supporters.

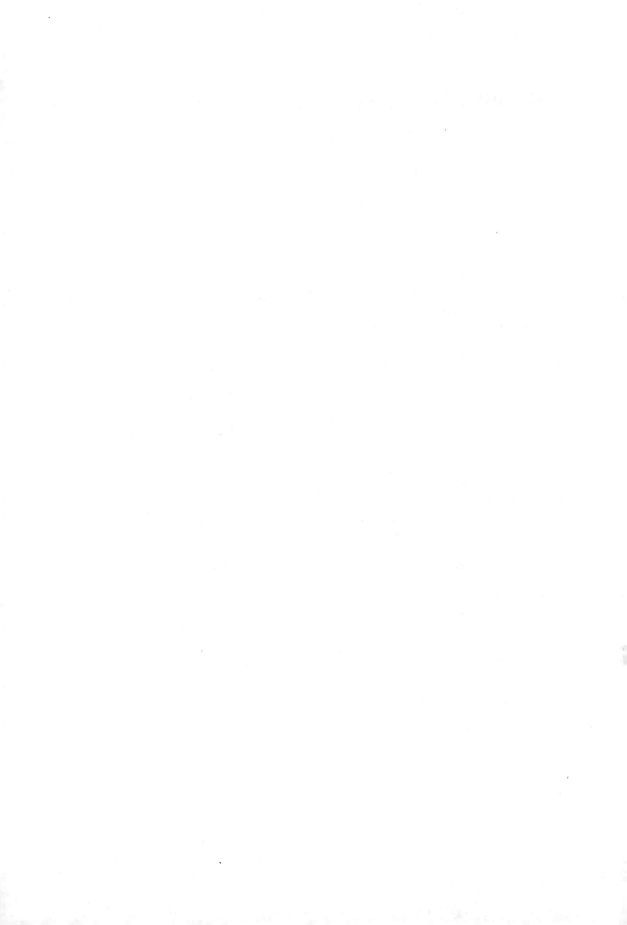

Breastfeeding for Public Health
A Resource for Community Healthcare Professionals

Alison Spiro

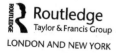
Routledge
Taylor & Francis Group

LONDON AND NEW YORK

Cover image: © Getty Images

First published 2022
by Routledge
4 Park Square, Milton Park, Abingdon, Oxon OX14 4RN

and by Routledge
605 Third Avenue, New York, NY 10158

Routledge is an imprint of the Taylor & Francis Group, an informa business

British Library Cataloguing-in-Publication Data
A catalogue record for this book is available from the British Library

Library of Congress Cataloging-in-Publication Data
Names: Spiro, Alison, author.
Title: Breastfeeding for public health : a resource for community healthcare professionals / Alison Spiro.
Description: Milton Park, Abingdon, Oxon ; New York, NY : Routledge, 2022. |
Includes bibliographical references and index. |
Identifiers: LCCN 2021040473 (print) | LCCN 2021040474 (ebook) |
ISBN 9780367689575 (hardback) | ISBN 9780367689568 (paperback) |
ISBN 9781003139775 (ebook)
Subjects: LCSH: Breastfeeding. | Infants--Nutrition.
Classification: LCC RJ216 .S656 2022 (print) | LCC RJ216 (ebook) |
DDC 613.2/69--dc23
LC record available at https://lccn.loc.gov/2021040473
LC ebook record available at https://lccn.loc.gov/2021040474

ISBN: 978-0-367-68957-5 (hbk)
ISBN: 978-0-367-68956-8 (pbk)
ISBN: 978-1-003-13977-5 (ebk)

DOI: 10.4324/9781003139775

Typeset in Times New Roman
by Taylor & Francis Books

Contents

Figures

Foreword

Breastmilk and breastfeeding can be regarded as the most important start that a baby has in her new life in the outside world. In the womb, she is held in the warmth and security of her mother's body, the pulsing umbilical cord providing the oxygen, nutrients and hormonal balance that creates and sustains life. She hears her mother's heart, her parents voices, she grows and develops until it is time to give birth. The natural start to life is to continue the nurturance, the development, attachment and love that breastfeeding can bring with its perfect combination of warm nutrients, water, antibodies and protection from illness. The importance of a safe and nurturing pregnancy is not contested, but breastfeeding by contrast has become an area of debate, often heated, about the choices a mother makes regarding infant feeding. In the UK the discussions and influences on these choices have eroded a baby's chances of being breastfed, especially beyond the first 8 weeks of life. The UK continues to have one of the lowest breastfeeding rates in the world, especially in terms of exclusive breastfeeding at 6 months and continued breastfeeding up to 2 years.

A parent's choice to breastfeed is influenced by multiple factors that Dr Spiro addresses in this text for health professionals. The text confronts the influence of the formula milk industry on parents' options, the role social and other media play in contributing to the often conflicting and confusing advice that parents receive from friends and family and from health professionals. She addresses the importance of time and space to breastfeed and what this means for new parents and how babies can benefit from that safe time and space being available to them.

Most importantly, the text is aimed at the health professional, especially health visitors, who can have an enormous impact and influence on parents' decisions about how to feed their baby. Dr Spiro brings together a wide range of evidence-based learning materials through each chapter of the book, based on her long-standing experience as a health visitor and breastfeeding consultant. Whilst breastfeeding is recognised in policy and by educators as an important part of the health visitor's role with parents (along with other professions including midwives, nursery nurses, lactation consultants and community practitioners) there are very few text books that address the ways in which they can support, promote and protect the breastfeeding environment for babies from a wide range of perspectives. The chapters address the health benefits and research underlying this, more recent discoveries such as the significance of the microbiome (gut flora) and its health promoting benefits, the issues surrounding the influence of the formula milk industry, the evolution of human milk banks and donor milk, as well as the practical tasks of observing and supporting breastfeeding.

The relationship between a mother and the health professional in the early days of life is most important. Dr Spiro has devoted much of the content of this book to enabling the professional to build a relationship of trust and empathy with parents, to become self-aware of their own experience and their communication style, to provide the support, encouragement and connection with local networks and community based services, enabling and empowering parents to breastfeed their baby with confidence.

The book provides an integration of research evidence, good practice and promotion of learning that will be vital to any health professional or student who is working with parents and infants, recognising the important part they can play in the support, promotion and protection of breastfeeding.

Professor Sally Kendall, MBE
PhD, RN, RHV
University of Kent

Acknowledgements

I would like to thank all my friends and colleagues who have made this book possible. They have encouraged me, been invaluable in reading chapters, sharing their knowledge and making positive comments.

In particular, Professor Sally Kendall for her insightful foreword and Patricia Wise who has commented on the text, using her extensive knowledge of the wider aspects of breastfeeding, and has been so helpful to me and generous with her time. I would like to thank my colleagues Tanya Dennis and Ursula Johnson for their encouragement and Julie Peris who has shared her expertise on practical issues and helped me find mothers who were kindly prepared to give me permission to use their photographs. Kathryn Stagg continues to give me so much information on the practicalities and emotional issues of breastfeeding twins and multiple babies. She has also generously shared her infographics, as have Heidi Hembury and Lucy Webber. Jenny Richardson gave me permission to include her very helpful line-drawing and Smita Hancelles shared the evidence she had on the close links between breastfeeding and maternal mental health.

Zainab Yate explained her work on breastfeeding aversion and agitation in Chapter 6 and has also given me invaluable help with my references. Cordelia Uys has kindly given me the use of her photographs as has Sherridan Stynest. Clare Castell and Olivia Vandyk from 'Blossom Antenatal' have agreed to me using one of their very informative slides.

I would like to thank all the parents who have given me permission to use their photographs and to Real Baby Milk for the use of some of their beautiful images.

I am very honoured that so many mothers were prepared for me to use their personal stories of the challenges that they faced with breastfeeding, some of which were physically and emotionally very difficult episodes in their lives.

Above all I would like to thank my husband Stephen for supporting and encouraging me in the last year, reading drafts, giving me useful comments and without whom this book would not have been possible.

Introduction: Inclusivity statement

This book supports feeding for all families and can be applied to all feeding parents. I recognise that there is variation in family structure and parenting styles. I will refer to parents as mothers and fathers but realise that some would prefer to be identified as female, male or non-binary. I will use the term 'breastfeeding' but am aware that some parents may prefer to use the term 'chest feeding'. I will be referring to the Equality Act 2010 (UK Government, 2010) which states that all families deserve culturally sensitive support suitable for their needs, irrespective of their age, race, marital status, sexual orientation, disability or gender reassignment.

1   Introduction

Why is breastfeeding in the UK still difficult?

Breastmilk gives a baby perfect nutrition; it is easy to digest and is uniquely designed for the age and gestation of an individual child, changing over time to ensure healthy growth and development. It is a living fluid, containing cells, antibodies, antibacterial and antiviral factors, stem cells, oligosaccharides, and a multitude of other ingredients offering a protective microbiome to the gut of the infant, and could be considered a type of personalised medicine.

Breastfeeding a baby is so much more than just a mechanical transfer of this amazing milk to babies and this book will address some of the wider social and cultural aspects of feeding. I will outline the physical advantages and the evidence that it protects parents' and babies' mental health.

Not being able to breastfeed can have a devastating effect on some mothers when they had planned to do so, which can leave them with deep feelings of loss and grief.[1] Unfortunately, in the UK so many women feel they have been let down by services which they believed in pregnancy would support them with breastfeeding after their babies were born. I am hoping this book will help to reverse this by giving community healthcare practitioners the self-awareness, information and practical skills they need to support women throughout their journey.

I will draw on some of my professional experience of 40 years of working as a health visitor in a North London borough as a generic and subsequently a specialist in breastfeeding, as well as an infant feeding lead in a local hospital.

What is the present global picture?

The World Health Organization (WHO) *Global Strategy for Infant and Young Child Feeding* was first published in 2003 and then reviewed in 2020.[2] It states that across the world only 40% of infants are exclusively breastfed for 6 months; and states that 820,000 children's lives globally could be saved if all children were optimally breastfed for up to 23 months. It aims to revitalise the efforts to promote, protect and support breastfeeding and builds on past initiatives such as the Innocenti Declaration (1990)[3] and the Baby Friendly Hospital Initiative (1991).[4] It calls on all governments to develop and implement policies and strategies to promote appropriate infant feeding. It recommends that the support given to mothers should be delivered by well-trained staff who can offer counselling skills and link with other support agencies in the community. Parents should be protected from the marketing of breastmilk substitutes by controlling advertising through legislation, as recommended in the WHO International Code.[5]

DOI: 10.4324/9781003139775-1

Mothers returning to work should be enabled to continue to breastfeed by having time and facilities to express and store their breastmilk.

What is happening in the UK?

The report of the World Breastfeeding Trends initiative (2016) assessed breastfeeding in the UK by looking at ten indicators, using an internationally recognised tool, through collaborating with government and third sector organisations. It concluded that 'despite the overwhelming evidence that breastfeeding protects and enhances health and wellbeing, it has become a contentious subject and progress in improving infant feeding through breastfeeding has been slow.'[6] It recommends policy action at all levels from communities, local government up to the NHS policymakers and national government. One of the indicators assessed the training that health professionalhs receive in breastfeeding and showed that in many cases it was insufficient, especially in some professional groups such as doctors, health visitors and dietitians.

Some improvements in health visiting training are beginning to happen through the work of the UNICEF UK Baby Friendly Initiative, with 72% of community NHS trusts now working towards accreditation. Universities training health visitors, however, have been slower to obtain this award, and still some who are newly qualified are starting their careers with little or no training in breastfeeding.

Following on from these international calls to protect and support breastfeeding, the UK decided to begin the process of Becoming Breastfeeding Friendly (BBF) in 2018, which is a global initiative led by Yale University, USA.[7] It is based on a 'gear model' which requires political action and commitment in order for the gears to turn and change to happen. A committee was formed of representatives from a government agency, professional bodies and third sector organisations, led by an academic department which carried out the research, and recommendations were drawn up to submit to government ministers. The Scottish and Welsh Governments published their policies and strategies from this initiative in 2019, and it is hoped that England will adopt theirs soon.

What is clear from these two initiatives is that more work needs to be done in the UK in training health visitors and some other professions in breastfeeding, if mothers are to get the consistent support they are asking for, enabling them to follow their chosen method of feeding their babies. It is hoped that this book will be helpful in outlining some of the knowledge and skills required to achieve this.

The Institute of Health Visiting recognises breastfeeding for its long-term impact on the health of an individual in its 'Vision for the Future' and as 'the biological norm'.[8] Formula milk supplementation should only be advised if it is medically indicated, if a mother wishes to breastfeed. Supporting breastfeeding is recognised by Public Health England as one of the health visitors' High Impact Areas.

Why is breastfeeding important for mothers and babies?

This book will discuss some of the rapidly growing evidence for the benefits that breastfeeding gives to mothers and children to build lifelong physical and mental health. Obesity presents the greatest burden of disease in Europe this century.[9] It has been shown that 1 in 3 children aged 6–9 years is obese, and over 50% of adults are overweight. It has been estimated that a child who has been breastfed is around 30%

less likely to suffer from obesity in childhood and later life. Breastfeeding has also been shown to offer some protection against other non-communicable diseases (NCDs) which include cardiovascular disease, diabetes, cancer and respiratory diseases which are the leading causes of death and disability in Europe.[10] Breastfeeding also improves IQ and school attendance, and research has shown that it is associated with better job prospects and higher incomes.[11] The emotional closeness the child develops with her mother when breastfeeding responsively helps to build a strong reciprocal relationship, aids brain development and increases feelings of trust, which in turn results in positive mental health outcomes.

Mothers also gain physical benefits from breastfeeding through gaining a reduced risk of breast and ovarian cancer, less osteoporosis, less heart disease and diabetes.[12] Despite these huge health benefits for mothers and children, and large savings to the health services, progress has been slow to establish national breastfeeding strategies across many countries in Europe, and at present there is very little governmental commitment to improving rates.

I will examine the current evidence and emerging research into the content of breastmilk, why it is so valuable for pre-term babies, describe how milk banks are evolving again in the UK and how mothers can donate milk to them.[13] I will be looking at some of the ways in which breastfeeding confers health benefits to mothers and babies, continuing long after breastfeeding finishes.

Breastmilk helps babies grow healthy microbiomes (gut flora), which impact on their future physical and psychological health and may make epigenetic (the way genes are expressed) changes in both mother and baby. Many researchers now see breastmilk as 'personalised medicine'[14] giving babies some lifelong protection from NCDs, and also some allergies and inflammatory conditions. I will also look at the work that has been done on the impact infant feeding has on the immune system and how milk shapes humans. Exclusive breastfeeding until 6 months of age gives babies optimum benefits, as recommended by WHO, the NHS and the Scientific Advisory Committee on Nutrition.

Babies and mothers develop close, loving relationships through the closeness of breastfeeding. Hormones such as oxytocin rise in mothers and babies during breast-feeding, which helps by relaxing them both into a sense of wellbeing and attachment. New and current research will be highlighted especially in the areas of relationships, brain growth, hormones and immunity. In order for mothers and children to enjoy these extensive benefits, many will need consistent practical and emotional support, especially in the early weeks after birth.

Why are community healthcare professionals in strong positions to offer support?

Health visitors and other community healthcare professionals in the UK provide a universal service and are able to visit all parents at home when their babies are 10–14 days old and during the first four years of the child's life. The long-term professional relationships they build with them of trust and empathy through a non-judgemental approach means their support can have profound impacts on the health and future life prospects for all members of the family. I will suggest ways in which investing *time* in the first few weeks of a baby's life can save *time* later on. The birth of a child heralds a very special, sensitive *time* for all new families, when they are beginning to adjust to life with a new baby both physically and psychologically.

Is there time for breastfeeding in the UK today?

I will look at *time* after the birth, when parents try to understand their babies' needs for food, comfort and reassurance, as well as looking after their own physical needs for rest, food and recuperation. In traditional societies and in some cultural groups in the UK, women are looked after by other women in their families, freed from domestic chores and so enabled to spend more time caring for their babies and adjusting emotionally to becoming parents.

Throughout the book I will reflect on my doctoral research in anthropology to look for possible insights I gained through interviewing mothers and use the themes of *time* and *place* for breastfeeding, which might be a helpful way to think about breastfeeding in the UK and to prioritise it in practice. I will also draw on my work as a volunteer breastfeeding counsellor for 30 years with a national charity, when I trained counsellors both locally and nationally.

Healthcare professionals may find it difficult to find the time to support parents with breastfeeding, but I suggest that time invested in supporting parents early after the birth of their babies will save time in the long term through building their self-confidence and preventing health and emotional problems.

Fathers and partners also go through this mental adjustment process at varying speeds and may need support too. I will be referring to breastfeeding parents and fathers, but I acknowledge that there can be variation in family structure and some parents may identify as non-binary. I also realise that some parents may prefer to use the term chest-feeding. The supportive partner of the breastfeeding person will always have a vital role to play in building confidence in her. Midwives and health visitors are in ideal positions to offer mothers, fathers and supportive partners timely and relevant breastfeeding support and information throughout the perinatal period.

Anthropologists call this time of adjustment to new family life a 'liminal period',[15] when parents are moving with their first babies from a time without children, to becoming a family with new responsibilities and concerns. This is a time which is 'betwixt and between', when many parents may require extra support and protection from the outside pressures of society. In some communities in the UK and in other countries in the world other women in the family protect a new mother from infections and malign influences by doing religious rituals, feeding the mother special foods and protecting her and her baby by keeping them apart from outsiders for the first month or six weeks after the birth.[16] Perhaps other families in Western societies believe they have moved away from practices like these, but it may be worth reflecting on them to see if we are giving new mothers in the UK enough space and support at this special time to adjust to their new lives. Women I interviewed wondered if there was time in modern day Britain for breastfeeding, which was perceived by some as being time-consuming, when they had household, social and work pressures. However, I will argue that breastfeeding can, in fact, save women time, such as the time needed to make up formula feeds, sterilise equipment and, most importantly, as babies are more likely to be healthy there may be fewer trips to the GP and fewer days off work.

This book also seeks to explore health visitors' time when they can support new families with feeding their babies. The profession currently suffers from reduced numbers in the workforce, with some having been redeployed in hospitals to assist with the COVID-19 crisis in 2020; thus, having enough time to spend with families can be a challenge, so effective interventions are crucial and any contact points with parents is planned, with active listening and reflection skills as essential components. I will look at the vital information and skills that it would be helpful for parents to understand, which may enable them to breastfeed for as long as they wish.

How does breastfeeding reduce social and health inequalities?

The recent report in 2020 by Sir Michael Marmot showed how the inequalities' gap has widened in the UK since his initial research in 2010, and how the COVID-19 crisis has worsened this divide.[17] Health visitors work with all communities in the UK, and 'proportionate universalism' is where universal services benefit everyone while putting in extra effort proportionate to need. Breastfeeding is key to improving lifelong physical and mental health and job opportunities.

Why is formula feeding considered 'normal' in the UK?

A father with a two-day-old baby whose wife was breastfeeding asked me on a hospital postnatal ward: 'When can my wife start "normal" feeding?'

Formula feeding has become the image that much of society in the UK sees when thinking about the common method of feeding babies, fanned by advertisements on television at peak family viewing times. In 1981 the World Health Organisation adopted the International Code of Marketing of Breastmilk Substitutes and afterwards adopted subsequent resolutions to address changes in marketing practices, scientific knowledge and questions of interpretation. Governments of the four nations of the UK have repeatedly endorsed the Code in order to protect breastfeeding but have not adopted it in its entirety. The aim of the Code is to contribute to the provision of safe and adequate nutrition for infants through the protection and promotion of breast-feeding and covers all breastmilk substitutes, feeding bottles and teats.

The 2005 resolution of the Code states: 'ensure that financial support and other incentives for programmes and health professionals working in infant and young child health do not create conflicts of interest'.[18] The UK government decided 40 years ago not to adopt the full WHO Code on the marketing of breastmilk substitutes, but instead to opt for a law forbidding the advertising and promotion of first milks, bottles and teats for babies under 6 months.

'Follow-on milks' for babies over this age can be advertised on television, advertising boards and in magazines, which often show images of babies looking less than 6 months being formula fed with bottles. I will suggest that these advertisements, shown on television at peak family times, serve to 'normalise' formula feeding in the UK. A study showed that immigrant mothers who come from breastfeeding cultures take only 18 months of living in the UK to think that formula feeding is the accepted way to feed babies in this country. I came across an example of this when an Indian mother, who had just given birth to her third baby here, said she had exclusively breastfed her first two children in India but: 'Mothers do not make enough milk for their babies in England'!

She decided to mix feed this baby with both breast and formula because she believed that she would not make enough milk in this country. Although she had a cultural preference to breastfeed, the effect of the *place*, now away from her country of birth, had a large impact on her decision making. New parents may think there is little difference between formula and breastmilk, through clever marketing. Perhaps concepts of place and social context do affect the perceived quantity and quality of the milk a mother makes.

Advertising of formula milk for babies of all ages appears in professional journals, and companies continue to sponsor some free health visitor training, gifts and awards. The arguments for continuing with these are that they serve to give health professionals information about products, although many professionals would prefer to access unbiased analysis of the ingredients in formula milk from nutritionists at the First Steps Nutrition Trust.

In 2020 the *British Medical Journal* editorial board decided to withdraw these advertisements and the Royal College of Paediatrics and Child Health sent guidance to their members to cease accepting sponsorship from companies which manufacture breastmilk substitutes. There is no doubt that the continuation of these advertisements sends messages to parents and the wider population that these products are almost as healthy as breastmilk.

Why do practical skills need to be embedded in practice?

Breastfeeding does not always come naturally to all women in the UK and health visitors have an important responsibility to teach these skills to mothers. The embodied knowledge needed to breastfeed has been lost in the last two generations and I will examine why this has happened. It may have begun in childhood when girls may have grown up owning dolls with bottles and watching women bottle feeding their babies in public places. Many women having their first babies have never seen a baby breastfeed, as many prefer to breastfeed at home behind closed doors. The bodily skills of how to hold and position babies and latch them on their breasts in the optimum way, may need to be to be learned in the way we learn to swim or ride a bike. Anthropologists call this 'bodily praxis', that is, the way we use our bodies to adopt certain skills, which then become embodied and 'second nature' or automatic. There are some essential skills which if adopted soon after the birth can determine the future breastfeeding trajectory for families and ensure that babies receive good milk transfer. Babies and mothers can change over time and sometimes subtle changes, or adjustments may be needed at a later stage.

These practical skills will be covered in depth and how they could be embedded in every health visitor's practice and guidelines, so that they become common place and used during every contact they have with mothers who wish to breastfeed. The last national survey that was carried out in 2010 showed that 80% of women in the UK start breastfeeding on the first day after their babies are born.[19]

This survey also showed that 74% of mothers stopped breastfeeding before they intended to and would have liked to carry on for longer. In this survey only 1–2% of mothers were exclusively breastfeeding at 6 months, which constitutes the lowest rate in the world.[20] The National Institute for Health and Care Excellence (NICE)[21] identified in the Postnatal Care Guideline that implementation of UNICEF Baby Friendly training should be a minimum standard for all professionals working with mothers and babies, but some health visitors have not yet reached this level. The 2015 national survey was cancelled by Public Health England, so it is difficult to know the present situation in the UK.

Universities training health visitors have been slow to achieve UNICEF UK Baby Friendly Initiative (BFI) accreditation (15%) compared with midwifery courses (47%).

If all universities were to achieve this standard, it would ensure that all newly qualified health visitors were able to support mothers with breastfeeding. It is good news that 72% of health visiting services in communities have achieved UNICEF BFI accreditation, showing that the profession is gradually becoming more informed about the practical skills needed to support breastfeeding.

Why are some health visitors and NHS trusts taking longer to embrace these, when breastfeeding is primary prevention par excellence? Is it because the time pressure of their other work, such as safeguarding children, feels overwhelming? Those professionals who have undergone breastfeeding training can demonstrate that they understand the importance of early skin-to-skin, optimum positioning and attachment, assessment of a breastfeed at their primary contact visit and how to give mothers the information they need on how to maintain their breastmilk supply. I will discuss that listening to parents' experience and concerns should come first before giving consistent, evidence-based breastfeeding information at the antenatal contact and first postnatal visit to give parents confidence in breastfeeding, and self-efficacy in their parenting skills.

Communication skills should begin by understanding our own beliefs and attitudes

Practitioners' self-awareness and opportunities to debrief their own personal past experiences in infant feeding can be very important for effective communication with parents. Health visitors are highly trained professionals in nursing, child development and public health and may feel that they have a wealth of knowledge to impart to parents, but a trusting, empathic relationship needs to be established first before any information can be given. Our attitudes can affect the way we present ourselves to others and parents can pick up on our body language through subtle gestures, as well as the way we listen to and respect their stories, enabling them to make their own decisions and gain confidence in breastfeeding.

Motivational interviewing skills may be helpful by establishing parents' goals and exploring with them ways to achieve them. These techniques will be described in more detail as a way to change attitudes and set goals through avoiding authoritarian, directive advice, with a focus on building self-efficacy to achieve their desired outcome.

Breastfeeding training should be ongoing and continued in supervision sessions, reflecting on how this is impacting on practice. All contacts concerning infant feeding need to include an element of listening to parents' stories, reflecting and summarising, being empathic, and through counselling skills helping mothers gain confidence in their breastfeeding ability. In this way parents can then see more clearly what areas they would like to change and begin to set their own goals.

Women who do not manage to reach their breastfeeding goals need empathy with any sense of grief and loss, in an attempt to help them overcome any guilt or shame and set goals for their future infant feeding. Unfortunately, many women find themselves in these situations where their hopes and plans have just not worked out, as Amy Brown said:

> Women need support, not just to breastfeed but to have real answers and to be able to talk through their experiences when it doesn't work out. That's what supporting and promoting breastfeeding also means and why we continue to call for investment for all women.[22]

Research in Australia identified an 'authentic presence' as someone who was 'being *there for me*' – either a health professional or lay supporter who showed empathy and listening skills as an effective supporter of mothers.[23] An empathic approach was also integral to an 'authentic presence', in which women feel that any help offered is supportive, rather than undermining, and is enhanced when the health professional or supporter listens in a warm and positive way. Health visitors are in a position to give this support to women, whatever their infant feeding outcomes may be, by being a warm, non-judgemental, empathic presence.

Does breastfeeding improve maternal mental health?

The simple answer to this is that, if breastfeeding goes well and women receive the support they need to meet their infant feeding goals, it can have a protective effect against postnatal depression.[24] Of course, there are degrees to the protection it offers and women's perceptions of their needs for support will vary.

Mothers often experience feelings of guilt if they do not, or find it too difficult to breastfeed, and may experience fear of failure. Fathers and partners can also suffer from some of these feelings, especially if they have not been able to give them adequate support. I will draw on some insights from a colleague's doctorate research on the subject of fathers and their transition to parenthood. Evidence exists that women's mental health is improved if they receive consistent, informed, accessible support, so achieving their infant feeding goals.

A recent blog written for the Institute of Health Visiting by a professor of child and adolescent psychiatry stated:

> Health visitors play a key role in supporting infant mental health during and after the COVID-19 crisis. Through their contact with parents, health visitors are well poised to raise awareness around support for parental wellbeing, responsive caregiving and early childhood development. Assessments of the basic psychosocial needs of the infant should include parental stress, anxiety and depression to identify those parents who are struggling. Services, where possible, should be sensitive to the financial and social needs of families, particularly those which have experienced bereavement related to COVID-19.[25]

A few mothers may have difficult physical and emotional experience of breastfeeding and may develop aversion. I will be exploring this in the context of current research.

Health visitors just weigh babies!

This may be a perception held by some mothers and other professionals who do not understand the wide scope of professional responsibilities and the abilities health visitors hold to undertake complex interventions with families. Mothers have traditionally seen health visitors at well baby clinics (before the COVID-19 pandemic), where they expected to have their babies weighed. These practices may have to change with social distancing and the emphasis will change and the focus will be on indicators of growth other than weight.

Health visitors may be criticised on social media that they are too quick to suggest supplementary feeds if babies are slow to gain weight, which may impact adversely on mothers' breastmilk supplies and confidence, heralding the end of breastfeeding. This could affect babies' and mothers' lifelong health outcomes.

How can health visitors give integrated support to parents?

Health visitors, nursery nurses, peer supporters, midwifery, paediatric and neonatal nurses can understand each other's roles, share the same policies on infant feeding and possibly train together. They can work jointly towards continuity and consistency of care and aim for mothers to receive less conflicting advice. I will share my experience here of working in hospital and community settings simultaneously, where I trained staff together, enabling staff to find common ground and build relationships.

Health visitors are more likely to signpost parents to the infant feeding team consisting of peer supporters, lactation consultants, breastfeeding counsellors and children's centre staff if they have built up relationships of trust. This can make their work more effective as parents receive more consistent support with breastfeeding.

There are networks of charities in the UK offering women free breastfeeding online and telephone support, through the National Breastfeeding Helpline, other helplines and social media, which are listed at the end of the book.

Some parents are presented with special challenges after they give birth such as being separated from their babies due to the need for either of them requiring medical attention. Babies born prematurely and those with congenital conditions may need to be admitted to a special care baby unit.

Parents expecting twins, or multiple births need special guidance on how they plan to feed their babies. Milk banks have an important role in supporting mothers and babies with breastfeeding. They can also serve to bridge the gap until babies are able and strong enough to breastfeed directly themselves.

In conclusion: can health visitors help to change public attitudes to breastfeeding?

Women support each other with breastfeeding all over the world! New mothers meet in families, villages, workplaces or other places such as community clinics or venues to share experiences and challenges. We need to recreate 'the village' in the UK, so women can meet and support each other more easily! In the present climate, these meeting places are often online, or on social media. An important part of health visitors' roles is to signpost them to antenatal breastfeeding workshops and postnatal breastfeeding support groups, and put them in touch with peer support programmes, evidenced-based apps, specialist Facebook groups, breastfeeding specialists, counsellors or International Board Certified Lactation Consultants (IBCLCs) for more complex issues.

I have written this book for practising, newly qualified, student community practitioners/health visitors, GPs, nursery nurses, peer supporters, practice nurses, children centre's staff and other practitioners, in an attempt to widen their knowledge base and suggest some practical and communication skills which may help when they support breastfeeding mothers. I am aware of the work pressures faced by health visitors and many of you are working with very large caseloads, often with increasing numbers of vulnerable families and safeguarding issues.

Health visitors are key to changing societal attitudes to breastfeeding, by supporting women who wish to breastfeed through giving them evidenced-based information, listening to their concerns, understanding and empathising with their feelings and enabling them to continue to feel good and confident.

Notes

1 Brown, A. (2019) *Why Breastfeeding Grief and Trauma Matter*. London: Pinter & Martin. Available at: www.pinterandmartin.com/why-breastfeeding-grief-and-trauma-matter

2 World Health Organization (WHO) (2003, 2020) *Global Strategy for Infant and Young Child Feeding*. Available at: www.globalbreastfeedingcollective.org/global-strategy-infant-and-young-child-feeding www.who.int/news-room/fact-sheets/detail/infant-and-young-child-feeding

3 UNICEF (2005) *Innocenti Declaration on the Protection, Promotion and Support of Breastfeeding*. Available at: www.unicef-irc.org/publications/434-1990-2005-celebrating-the-innocenti-declaration-on-the-protection-promotion-and-support.html

4 WHO (1991) *Ten Steps to Successful Breastfeeding*. Available at: www.who.int/activities/promoting-baby-friendly-hospitals/ten-steps-to-successful-breastfeeding

5 UNICEF (1981) *The International Code of Marketing of Breastmilk Substitutes: Baby Friendly Initiative*. Available at: www.unicef.org.uk/babyfriendly/baby-friendly-resources/international-code-marketing-breastmilk-substitutes-resources/the-code/

6 About WBTi (2016) *Breastfeeding Trends (UK)*, 13 September. Available at: https://ukbreastfeeding.org/about/

7 Yale School of Public Health (2018) *Becoming Breastfeeding Friendly: A Guide to Global Scale Up*. Available at: https://publichealth.yale.edu/bfci/

8 See https://ihv.org.uk/our-work/our-vision/

9 Rito *et al.* (2019) 'Association between characteristics at birth, breastfeeding and obesity in 22 countries: The WHO European Childhood Obesity Surveillance Initiative – COSI 2015/2017', *Obesity Facts*. https://pubmed.ncbi.nlm.nih.gov/31030194/

10 WHO (2021) *About Child and Adolescent Health*. Available at: www.euro.who.int/en/health-topics/Life-stages/child-and-adolescent-health/about-child-and-adolescent-health

11 Victora, C. G. *et al.* (2015) 'Association between breastfeeding and intelligence, educational attainment, and income at 30 years of age: A prospective birth cohort study from Brazil', *The Lancet Global Health*, 3(4), pp. 199–205.

12 Chowdhury, R. *et al.* (2015) 'Breastfeeding and maternal health outcomes: A systematic review and meta-analysis', *Acta Paediatrica (Oslo, Norway: 1992)*, 104(467), pp. 96–113.

13 Hearts Milk Bank (2020) *About Us – Hearts Milk Bank (2020)* Available at: https://heartsmilkbank.org/about-us/

14 Rollins, N. and Doherty, T. (2019) 'Improving breastfeeding practices at scale', *The Lancet Global Health*, 7(3), pp. e292–e293.

15 Turner, V. (1969) 'Rite of passage and anti-structure'. *Encyclopedia Britannica*. Available at: www.britannica.com/topic/rite-of-passage

16 Moran, V. H. and Dykes, F. (eds) (2005) *Maternal and Infant Nutrition and Nurture: Controversies and Challenges*. London: Quay Books.

17 Marmot, M. (2020) 'Health equity in England: The Marmot Review 10 years on', *British Medical Journal*, 368, p. m693.

18 WHA Resolution 58.32 (2005). Infant and young child nutrition: The Forty-first World Health Assembly. Available at: www.nationalestillfoerderung.de/images/who-resolutionen/wha_res_58_32.pdf

19 Infant Feeding Survey – UK, 2010 (2012) NHS Digital. Available at: https://digital.nhs.uk/data-and-information/publications/statistical/infant-feeding-survey/infant-feeding-survey-uk-2010

20 Rollins, N. C. *et al.* (2016) 'Why invest, and what it will take to improve breastfeeding practices?', *The Lancet*, 387(10017), pp. 491–504.

21 National Institute for Health and Care Excellence (NICE) (2006) *Overview: Postnatal Care up to 8 Weeks after Birth: Guidance*. Available at: www.nice.org.uk/guidance/cg37

22 Brown, A. (2020) 'Supporting those who haven't been able to breastfeed'. Institute of Health Visiting. Available at: https://ihv.org.uk/news-and-views/voices/supporting-those-who-havent-been-able-to-breastfeed/ (Accessed: 13 July 2021).

23 Schmied, V. *et al.* (2011) 'Women's perceptions and experiences of breastfeeding support: A metasynthesis', *Birth*, 38(1), pp. 49–60.

24 Borra, C., Iacovou, M. and Sevilla, A. (2015) 'New evidence on breastfeeding and post-partum depression: The importance of understanding women's intentions', *Maternal and Child Health Journal*, 19(4), pp. 897–907.

25 Stein, A. (2020) 'Health visiting 2020: Helping babies to thrive, not just survive through the COVID pandemic', Institute of Health Visiting. Available at: https://ihv.org.uk/news-and-views/voices/health-visiting-2020-helping-babies-to-thrive-not-just-survive-through-the-cov id-pandemic/

2 Why does breastfeeding matter to babies, mothers and society?

The evidence that breastfeeding confers lifelong health to mothers and babies and improves public health, is now extensive.[1] Knowledge of this is essential for all community practitioners, to enable you to answer questions parents may ask and direct resources to address local health needs. These only need to be communicated to parents at a time appropriate to their situation, bearing in mind that it may lead to feelings of guilt if breastfeeding does not work for them, or is not socially acceptable in their families or communities around them. Although most parents today in the UK have heard the 'breast is best' message, rather than breastfeeding is the biologically normal way to feed babies, many do not think that it is achievable, convenient or appropriate for them and their babies, as formula feeding may be thought as more modern and reliable. Sensitivity to their feelings, their experiences of infant feeding and existing knowledge is essential, before any of the following research is shared. In this chapter, I will outline some of the latest evidence, covering the main areas where babies who are not breastfed may be disadvantaged and will draw on review articles and meta-analyses when possible, and on the very important Lancet Series published in 2016, to which I will be referring throughout this chapter:

> Breastfeeding is a child's first inoculation against death, disease, but also their most enduring investment in physical, cognitive, and social capacity.[2]

Although most babies in the UK are formula fed, and often appear to thrive, they may live with the consequences of not being breastfed for the rest of their lives.

Why is breastfeeding important for babies' health?

Many people in the UK have some understanding that breastfeeding gives babies protection against infectious diseases, although a few may think, falsely, that this is only important in developing countries. In the UK, the numbers of infants and children, mostly formula fed, who present at GP surgeries and A&E departments with common infections, cause a huge financial burden on the UK Government's purse. If mothers breastfeed their infants exclusively for the first four months, estimated savings of over £12 million could be made annually[3] (based on the value of the pound in 2012; it is likely to be considerably more in 2021).

It is clear that putting resources into supporting women to breastfeed successfully would be hugely cost effective for the NHS, as well as preventing the distress and pain felt by a mother who has a bad experience of breastfeeding.[4]

DOI: 10.4324/9781003139775-2

Anecdotally, when I was working in a GP practice in an outer London borough, the doctors told me that they rarely saw the breastfed babies (apart from at check-ups) in the surgery, because they were hardly ever unwell!

What is the evidence that breastfeeding protects against infectious diseases?

There is now a strong evidence base that breastfeeding helps to protect against the incidence of many of the common diseases of childhood, such as diarrhoea, respiratory infections and ear infections, which can cause infants and young children to be admitted to hospital.

Breastfeeding can prevent 72% of hospital admissions for young infants throughout the world.[5] Diarrhoeal disease kills 5 million children a year in the developing world and the risk of dying is reduced by 20-fold in breastfed children. Similarly, breastfeeding helps to protect babies against respiratory infections, including reducing hospital admissions across all countries.

Ear infections are a common cause of crying and unhappiness in babies and breastfeeding helps to reduce their frequency and severity. There is also consistent evidence on the protection it gives against acute otitis media in the first 2 years of life.[6]

As we all know, when working with families, these diseases are very common and do not only cause infants to become very unwell, sometimes rapidly, but can also lead to families feeling very anxious and distressed. Exclusive breastfeeding will give infants the best protection, but any amount of breastmilk will help, to a lesser extent, in a dose-related way.

A meta-analysis of four randomised controlled trials of necrotising enterocolitis showed that babies who received breastmilk showed a reduction of 58% in the incidence of this bowel condition affecting sick and premature infants, who may have required major surgery to remove sections of their bowels, which carries a high risk of fatality in all settings.[7]

Another meta-analysis of six studies showed a 36% reduction in sudden infant death syndrome (SIDS)[8] in infants who had been breastfed. Breastfeeding could help to avoid these devastating events for some families, but any communication of this information needs to be done at an appropriate time and very sensitively.

In 2020 the Royal College of Paediatrics and Child Health released a report on the State of Child Health and Wellbeing in the UK. This covered asthma, diabetes and epilepsy, as well as the risk factors for poor health such as obesity, child deaths and the low rate of breastfeeding. It demonstrated the urgent need to respond to the large health inequalities between rich and poor communities in the UK, with infant mortality being more than twice as high in the lowest compared with the highest socio-economic groups.[9]

The mother will pass specific antibodies to her child in her breastmilk, to any infections she has encountered. If she is currently suffering herself from symptoms, any pathogens she inhales or ingests will be picked up through her broncho-mammary pathway and within hours her milk will be giving her baby some protection. You will find that if a whole family is suffering from a respiratory infection, the breastfed baby is likely to remain healthy, or only suffer from very mild symptoms. This protection for babies is the reason it is so important that mothers continue to breastfeed while they are suffering from infections.

New research from Birmingham has demonstrated the activation of babies' T cells and regulatory immune cells in response to maternal cells in breastmilk in the first 3 months of life.[10]

Is there evidence that breastfeeding helps to protect against non-communicable diseases?

Non-communicable diseases present a growing burden of ill health across the UK today, such as obesity, diabetes, cardio-vascular disease, cancer and auto-immune diseases. These disproportionately affect those living in areas of social deprivation. A review which clarified the link between the prevention of auto-immune diseases and breastfeeding found that having been breastfed was associated with lower incidence of diabetes, coeliac disease, multiple sclerosis and asthma. The mechanism whereby this happens is not fully clear but the authors suggest that the protection breastmilk affords against early infections, is through its anti-inflammatory properties, antigen-specific tolerance and the way it regulates the infant's microbiome.[11]

Does breastfeeding protect against childhood obesity?

Obesity is a huge, growing public health problem in the UK and in many countries across the world. It is now an increasingly common cause of mortality and morbidity in adults and children and underlies some of the main causes of ill health and admissions to hospital. Childhood obesity is estimated to affect one child in five in this country and measures taken so far do not seem to be affecting the rates.

You are probably finding in your practice that, once a child becomes identified as being overweight, it is difficult to change eating practices. Breastfeeding provides a preventative approach to a child gaining too much weight, so enabling mothers to breastfeed for as long as they wish is likely to have an impact on preventing so many children from becoming overweight. The WHO European Childhood Obesity Study (COSI) looked at the prevalence of obesity in 22 countries in 6–9-year-old children, and confirmed the beneficial effects of breastfeeding, with the highest level of obesity found in children who had never been breastfed.

Unless this is tackled soon, these children will carry burdens of risk of disease through into adult life. There is evidence from meta-analyses that the risk of a child becoming overweight or obese is reduced by breastfeeding. This effect is dependent on the duration of breastfeeding – the longer a child is breastfed, the lower the risk.

How does breastfeeding help to protect children against obesity?

The mechanism of how this happens is not yet fully understood, but you will notice how those who were exclusively breastfed for 6 months and then breastfed alongside solid foods are less likely to be overweight at one year. One explanation might be that human milk establishes a healthy gut microbiome and that hormones and fatty acids are likely to have a programming role in maintaining a normal weight in later life. Non-breastfed babies will not have had this developmental programming so may be more susceptible to environmental pressures to become obese.[12]

We know that breastmilk changes during a feed with the protein and fat content rising with the 'let down' and the mother having surges of oxytocin in response to her baby. Babies respond to these changes in milk ingredients; in hot weather they will have short, frequent feeds to satisfy their thirst with more watery foremilk, and when having growth spurts will have longer, frequent feeds to give them more hindmilk and calories. Once their hunger or thirst has been satisfied, they come off the breast or fall asleep as they react to this feeling of fullness and satisfaction; this may lead to better appetite control which may be one of the mechanisms that may help to prevent obesity in later life. A baby who is well positioned and attached to the breast will get good milk transfer and will control the volume and content of the breastmilk he/she receives.

Unfortunately, there has been misunderstanding of the research done in the 1980s which recommended that babies who are well attached will breastfeed and transfer milk efficiently. Babies take a variable length of time to transfer this breastmilk and, wrongly, people have imposed specific timings that babies need to feed on the first breast. We need to trust babies to take what they need, let them finish feeding themselves. Their bodies tell them what they need!

Breastfeeding babies with no time schedules will respond to their feeding cues and ensure they get everything they need if they are feeding well. Babies learn to recognise when their stomachs are full and stop feeding, so are less likely to over-feed and less likely to become obese.

When breastfeeding, infants learn this control over their appetites by coming off the breast when their stomachs are full, and there is some evidence that if they are bottle-fed breastmilk, or formula milk this appetite control mechanism may not develop so effectively. A study of 2,553 mother–infant dyads in the USA showed that babies who were exclusively breastfed directly at 3 months had lower BMIs at 12 months; but those given breastmilk from a bottle were not so well protected, and those supplemented with formula or exclusively formula-fed had the highest obesity rates.[13] Responsive bottle feeding may help this 'full stomach' response to develop, as the baby has more control over the flow of the milk and the volume consumed. The baby is invited to take the teat into his/her mouth and rather than tipping the bottle towards vertical during feeding it is kept horizontal; this enables the baby to control the flow of milk and finish feeding when full.

The only exceptions to this may be if babies have special health problems which I will deal with in another chapter.

Does breastfeeding offer protection against obesity in later life?

Evidence from 113 studies shows that breastfeeding not only reduces the chances of a child becoming obese by 26%[14] but also there is good evidence from three moderate quality meta-analyses suggesting that the risk of obesity is also *reduced in later life*. In the first, Harder[15] reviewed 17 studies and concluded that every month of breastfeeding was associated with a 4% decrease in risk. In the second, Arenz[16] reviewed nine studies, and found that breastfeeding appears to have a small but consistent protective effect against obesity. In the third, Owen[17] reviewed 61 studies, and again found a reduced risk of obesity in later life even when confounding variables such as parental obesity, maternal smoking and social class were taken into account.

It is thought that breastfeeding also helps children regulate their food intake and energy balance through the hormones and biological properties in the breastmilk, which may assist in 'programming' an individual to have a 25% lower risk of becoming obese in later life.[18]

Why do children who were breastfed choose healthier diets?

This COSI study also found that children who had been breastfed were more likely to choose a diet high in fruit and vegetables than those who had been formula fed. The reasons for this are not fully understood, but it is thought that when infants and children are breastfed, they taste their mothers' diets in their milk, which may help them adjust to different flavours when complementary foods are introduced.

What can the UK do to address the problem of childhood obesity?

I am surprised that the UK Government agencies so far do not seem to have taken this protective effect into account when planning the obesity strategy. There is now compelling evidence that breastfeeding offers children a reduction in the chances of becoming obese by 25–30% through both the balance of the ingredients of breastmilk itself, as well as babies controlling their own milk intake, and stopping feeding at the breast when satisfied when directly breastfed from their mothers.

The WHO has called for curbs to be made on the marketing of breastmilk substitutes as an important step towards tackling this obesity epidemic.[19] Our breastfeeding rates in the UK continue to be low with only 1% of children being breastfed exclusively up to 6 months.[20] 74% of mothers start breastfeeding and most would have liked to continue for longer than they did but feel let down by the lack of support from professionals, families and friends. This leads to a large number of new mothers in our society feeling guilty that they have been unable to give their children the best start to their lives. I will discuss this further in the chapter on maternal mental health and the potentially devastating effect on mothers of not being supported to feed their babies in the way they wished.[21]

What other non-communicable diseases of childhood can be reduced by breastfeeding?

There has been shown in two studies that the associated risk of a child developing type 2 diabetes is 14% lower in those who had been breastfed.[22]

It has also been shown that breastfeeding for 9.6 months or longer has a protective effect against developing childhood leukaemia, and for neuroblastoma to a lesser extent, but there was no evidence for other childhood cancers.[23]

Exclusive breastfeeding provides a reduced risk of developing asthma in children up to the age of six and a degree of protection after this age, which was more pronounced in those who were atopic.[24] Research from Canada showed that exclusive breastfeeding for 6 months, with no supplementary formula feeds gave infants of asthmatic mothers a protection against asthma of 62%, independent of smoking, education and other risk factors. Children who received partial breastfeeding with additional foods were found to have a 37% reduction in asthma, but if supplemented with formula there was no significant protection. Breastfeeding appeared to have a protective effect against wheezing in a dose-dependent way among infants born to mothers with asthma.[25] The evidence is not so strong on the protective effect of breastfeeding against eczema and allergic rhinitis, but controlling for variables is difficult here with many environmental factors and confounding variables.

Exclusive breastmilk feeding for at least the first three months leads to reduced cholesterol levels in late adolescence, with a healthier lipid profile, which is likely to lead to long-term benefits for cardiovascular health.[26]

Breastfeeding has been associated with a reduced risk of dental malocclusion. However, normal dental hygiene should be observed because once teeth have erupted, they are vulnerable to caries and should be cleaned with fluoride toothpaste twice a day.

The evidence base is now extensive on the protective effect breastfeeding affords against these diseases and new research findings are coming to light every month.

Do adults have better job prospects if they were breastfed?

A wider global view, where exclusive breastfeeding is more common, might shed more light on the role of breastfeeding in increasing the child's attainments and future job prospects. A study in Brazil was carried out over 30 years suggesting an effect of breastfeeding on intelligence, school attainment, and adult earnings.[27] They compared children who were never breastfed with those who were ever breastfed and the length of period of breastfeeding. The cohort was followed up into adolescence and adulthood, finding that there was an increase in IQ of 3–5 points in those who were breastfed. The adults who were breastfed as babies had better job prospects.

Does breastfeeding help children's physical fitness?

The physical fitness of over 5,000 children aged 7 who were breastfed exclusively for 6 months was shown to be raised by 10–40% in high performance tests.[28] After the researchers had adjusted for confounding factors, both boys and girls in the group who had been breastfed had more overall body strength and cardio-respiratory fitness. More studies are needed to confirm these findings, but it demonstrates the wider, long-term health implications of early infant feeding.

Does breastfeeding benefit mothers' health too?

It is less well known in society that breastfeeding improves women's health for the rest of their lives and every month of doing it exclusively will make a difference!

Mothers who breastfeed for up to one year have been shown in six studies to have lower incidences of type 2 diabetes.[29] The risks of invasive breast cancer are also reduced with parity and duration of breastfeeding with an estimate that for every 12 months of breastfeeding the risk is reduced by 6%, when confounding factors have been taken into account.[30]

Exclusive breastfeeding over several months has been shown to be associated with a 30% reduction in the incidence of ovarian cancer in 41 studies.[31] This could be associated with the fact that women who predominantly breastfeed have longer times of lactational amenorrhoea (lack of menstruation) which affects their fertility and lengthens the interval between pregnancies, enabling them to space their children.

Some women in your case load may have cultural or religious reasons why they do not want to use medical forms of contraception and having fewer children by exclusively breastfeeding, before their periods return, may benefit the health of other members of the family, as well as the family purse. The contraceptive effect relies on frequent stimulation of the breasts through breastfeeding exclusively day and night, so the hormones of lactation delay the return of ovulation and menstruation. Once the woman's periods return, or when her baby starts to sleep through the night, or she offers other food or milk to her baby, or she is unwell, or is prescribed antibiotics, the contraceptive effect may be lost. The NHS has some clear guidance on this method of spacing children (www.nhs.uk/conditions/contraception/natural-family-planning/).

Breastfeeding appears to improve mothers' bone density and *reduce* their chances of developing **osteoporosis** in later life. Although lactating women may lose more bone mineral content than non-lactating women in the first 6 months postpartum, after stopping breastfeeding women who had lactated gained significantly more bone content than women who had formula-fed their babies.

If you are able to support mothers to breastfeed their babies exclusively for 6 months or longer, it will reduce their chances of getting type 2 diabetes, breast or ovarian cancer and osteoporosis or other autoimmune diseases such as rheumatoid arthritis and will improve their long-term health prospects.

The time and effort you invest in supporting mothers in the first few months of their babies' lives will pay off, as they will become more confident as mothers, protect their own health, build their self-efficacy and close relationships with their children. Both infants' and their mothers' health will have beneficial long-term health outcomes. This is primary prevention in its purest form, a priority for all health visitors, and will improve community health and save NHS resources by reducing the need for GP consultations and hospital treatment.

What do we know about the wonders of breastmilk itself?

Breastmilk is human milk for human babies! It is a dynamic, living fluid which contains thousands of different molecules, growth factors, hormones, microorganisms and cells, which work together to provide the human baby with all the ingredients necessary to grow and develop normally. Many of its components have only recently been discovered, leaving the tantalising possibility that more remain and the functions of many remain unknown.

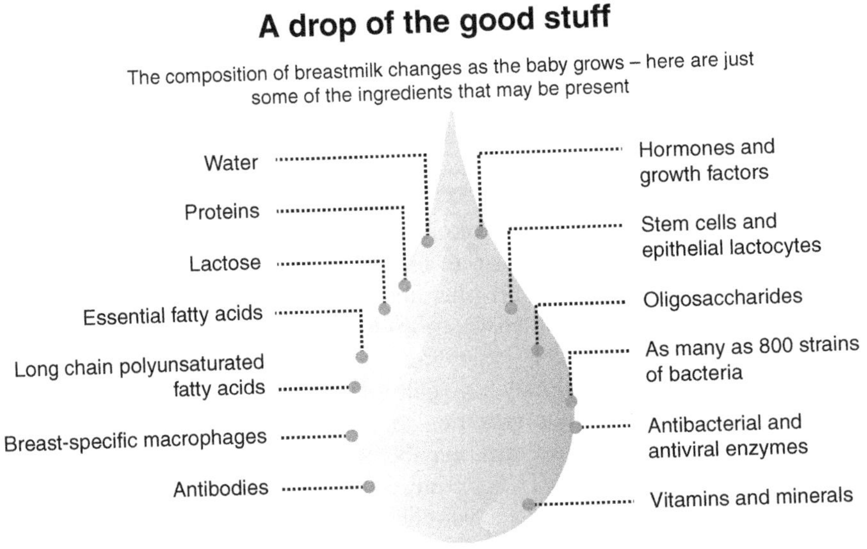

A drop of the good stuff

The composition of breastmilk changes as the baby grows – here are just some of the ingredients that may be present

Water

Proteins

Lactose

Essential fatty acids

Long chain polyunsaturated fatty acids

Breast-specific macrophages

Antibodies

Hormones and growth factors

Stem cells and epithelial lactocytes

Oligosaccharides

As many as 800 strains of bacteria

Antibacterial and antiviral enzymes

Vitamins and minerals

Figure 2.1 Breastmilk contains a multitude of human and non-human cells as well as nutrients, hormones and other immune system-related components (Shenker, 2019).

What does breastmilk contain?

Breastmilk contains the perfect macronutrients for babies and these constituents change over time to meet their needs as they develop and grow. It is 'bioavailable', meaning that it is easy for babies' immature digestive systems to absorb the human milk proteins, carbohydrates, long-chain fatty acids, hormones, bifidus factor, immunoglobulins, growth factors, stem cells and specific micro-organisms which help to fight infections. Formula milk in the UK is primarily made from cow's milk, which is absorbed more slowly and uses more energy to do so and is more likely to cause colic and reflux. This will feed the baby's body but does not give the same protection against disease. The mother's breasts seem to know the age of her baby, by producing the perfect nutrition, whether the baby is premature, one day or one year old!

Breastmilk also contains living cells, more similar to blood than what we normally think of as milk! It has white cells, called macrophages, which swallow up harmful bacteria and viruses, as well as antibacterial and antiviral factors and antibodies. Over 800 different strains of beneficial bacteria have been identified in human milk, along with oligosaccharides (milk sugars) which are thought to feed these bacteria and maintain the baby's microbiome. Over 300 ingredients have been identified in breastmilk to date, but it is likely there are hundreds more which we have yet to identify. The oligosaccharides in breastmilk cannot be absorbed by the baby but also have an anti-infective property function to block antigens from attaching to the walls of the baby's gut, which seems to be particularly effective against bacteria that cause pneumonia and sepsis.[32] Antibodies can be found in breastmilk itself as well as in the cells and are targeted against infectious agents in the environment, so offering the baby protection.

Why is colostrum so valuable?

Colostrum is probably the most important milk the baby will ever have. It is made in the mother's breast from 16 weeks of pregnancy and provides a dense, energy-rich food for babies in the first 2–3 days after birth in just a few millilitres per feed. It coats the inside of the baby's gut and is sometimes known as a protective layer of 'white paint'. It is made of white blood cells, many of which are macrophages which engulf and absorb harmful organisms and also manufacture lactoferrin, an iron-binding protein which not only helps the baby to absorb and store iron, but at the same time prevents the growth of harmful bacteria such as E. coli and some Staphylococcus species and fungal infections like Candida.

It also contains lysozyme, an enzyme which has antibacterial and antiviral effects by attacking their cell walls. Both lactoferrin and lysozyme continue to be present in transitional milk too (the milk mothers make in the first six weeks, which is a mixture of colostrum and mature milk), and continue to be found in mature milk; their concentrations increase when babies get older and become mobile, helping them to cope with new pathogens.

Colostrum is usually made in small volumes which is perfect for the new-born baby's stomach, which is about the size of a small cherry after birth. Some mothers like to collect or 'harvest' their colostrum towards the end of pregnancy and freeze it as a back-up if their babies are separated from them, if they have gestational diabetes, or their babies take time to latch on the breast. There are helpful videos on collecting colostrum in pregnancy on YouTube.

Broncho-mammary pathway

Mothers often worry whether it is safe for them to breastfeed if they have colds or influenza, but we can reassure them that it is not only safe, but desirable to do so, because their immune system works to protect their babies through their breastmilk. If a mother inhales a pathogen, then the lymph nodes in her lungs manufacture specially sensitised lymphocytes which migrate to her breasts and make specific antibodies against that bacteria or virus.[33] In the current COVID-19 pandemic, research in Holland has shown that women who have suffered from the disease are making antibodies to coronavirus in their breastmilk. This Dutch team is investigating whether these antibodies could help to protect vulnerable people from the COVID-19 virus, possibly in the form of ice cubes made from pasteurised donor milk. It is thought that after drinking this breastmilk, the antibodies attach themselves to the surface of mucous membranes and attack the virus before it enters the person's body.

How does breastfeeding impact babies' brains?

The fats in breastmilk are long-chain fatty acids that are specifically suited to help the maturation of babies' nerve cells in the brain and spinal cord by 'firing' the synapses between the cells. These are very diverse, supporting the complexity of the large human brain. Cow's milk does not contain enough of these (cows have relatively smaller brains!) and formula milk made from this needs to be supplemented from other sources, often fish by-products. Many of these components have only recently been discovered and probably hundreds more will be found in the next few years. Breastmilk also contains stem cells and the function of these is not well understood, but they have been found in the brains and kidneys of infants.

Mothers' and babies' bodies and brains communicate together through breastfeeding! Babies and mothers make oxytocin (the 'love' hormone) in their pituitary glands, especially when they are in skin-to-skin contact or breastfeeding. This closeness helps babies' emotional centres in their brains develop and, when fed responsively from the breast or bottle, feelings of trust develop in the baby that the parent will respond to their feeding cues; the mother feels relaxed and has a sense of well-being. Sleep cycles may be established through the differing, diurnal levels of cortisol in breastmilk, but this is not fully understood yet.

Does breastfeeding raise children's IQs?

The discussion about the link between breastfeeding and intelligence is contentious, because of potential confounding factors. Some people argue that the most important factors determining how well children perform at school and beyond are because of the stimulation a child receives at home and the importance a family places on education. Perhaps it is difficult in high-income countries to separate the two because the mothers who are most likely to breastfeed are those who have received education themselves beyond the age of 18 years. Headlines in 2017 in the public press attracted public attention by suggesting that breastfeeding did not affect intelligence. It was based on the longitudinal infant cohort study 'Growing up in Ireland' which identified families from the Child Benefit Register and parents were asked to report retrospectively. Rates of exclusive and partial breastfeeding at that time were very low. The length of breastfeeding was reported by mothers retrospectively, and parents and teachers reported with standardised assessments of the children's behaviours, so making correlations with how a child was fed and future intelligence was difficult. Other observational studies however, showed higher school attainment in five cohorts from high- and middle-income countries and consistent effects of an IQ rise of three points in children who had been breastfed.[34] Considering and controlling for confounding factors, such as the education of the parents, age and social standing, in any study are essential if any valid conclusions are to be made.

Breastmilk itself contains essential building blocks for the baby's brain at each stage of the child's development. In a study of 133 children between 10 months and 4 years, MRI scans showed that those who had been breastfed had increased white matter development in several regions of their brains, demonstrating they had an increase in healthy neural growth, which might impact on their development and future IQ.[35]

Mother's breast to infant gut microbiome

We are beginning to understand that breastmilk itself feeds the good bacteria which line the infant's gut to give him/her healthy and diverse microbiomes. They inactivate harmful bacteria and viruses, influencing babies to build their own immune systems and setting up prospects for lifelong health.

Recent evidence has indicated that there is close communication between the mother's breast and her infant's gut bacteria – 56% of the cells in the human body are microbial cells, with 2 million genes in total! They have a vital role in maintaining health and protecting the gut lining against invading microorganisms.

Early research into the breast and gut microbiome is beginning to explain how the baby gets protection against infections, but still only a few of the many components of human milk have been identified. Some researchers think that the bacteria in mothers' milk are carried from their intestines by dentritic cells, which send out projections into their intestinal epithelium and take up bacteria from their gut lumens. These cells then communicate with gut lymphocytes and travel through the lymphatic system to other mucosal surfaces including the lactating mammary glands where they are secreted into the breastmilk. So, the breast itself has its own microbiome, in which is a complex ecosystem of bacteria, viruses, and fungi. The breast should be seen as an immune organ, which was its only function before it evolved to provide nutrition as well, although it is never listed as such in medical textbooks.

After a baby has had a feed of breastmilk, these bacteria, especially bifido-bacterium, which is the dominant species, and other organisms act in the babies' guts after they have passed from their stomachs to their small intestines. The special sugars in breastmilk are called human milk oligosaccharides (HMOs) which are not absorbed by the infant, but are thought to feed the good bacteria in the gut. This microbiome forms a protective covering inside the baby's gut, which stops harmful bacteria, viruses and other proteins from entering their bodies, which are then excreted in the stools. The Teddy Study followed 903 infants from 3 to 46 months and showed that breastmilk, either exclusive or partial, was the most significant factor associated with microbiome structure, but exclusive breast-feeding had the greatest impact.[36] This immune protection covers the time when the baby is most vulnerable and the immune system is immature, from the early period after birth, throughout childhood and beyond, even after breastfeeding has ceased. The composition of the breastmilk microbiome changes over months and years, and work is ongoing to understand the impact this has on the developing gut. It seems to have an important protective function in premature babies, who have particularly immature guts; breastmilk helps to seal gaps in the lining, preventing pathogenic bacteria from entering his/her body and reducing the likelihood of necrotising-enterocolitis (NEC). The mother may also benefit by having her immune system stimulated which seems to help her postnatal recovery, but this has yet to be substantiated. Formula fed babies have different gut bacteria which do not give them as much protection from pathogens.

How is new research beginning to explain the complexity of the biological processes?

There is emerging evidence on the mechanisms whereby breastfeeding not only affects the infants' gut microbiota composition, but may also link with the way their genes are expressed. This may begin to throw light on how it gives some protection against these infectious and non-communicable diseases that I have described above. Interestingly, the gut microbiota in infants are influenced by the way they receive the breastmilk. Those who have been breastfed directly from the breast have more diverse good bacteria in their guts, than those fed expressed milk. The conclusion drawn from this finding is that bacteria in the baby's oral cavity may affect the breast and the good bacteria found in breastmilk which in turn affects their microbiomes.[37]

Researchers have found that nutrition in early life has a role in modulating gene expression which is called 'nutrigenetics',[38] and the way nutrition affects the child's 'epigenetic' profile. Epigenetics literally means the 'top of genetics' referring to way genes are expressed, without influencing the gene sequence, but can be passed on to the next generation.

New research has found a link between epigenetic mechanisms and the programming of asthma, which potentially may be linked to the interaction with the intestinal microbiota. Other perinatal environmental factors as well as breastfeeding are also believed to have a role here which may influence the gut flora, including caesarean section, perinatal stress, probiotics and antibiotics.

This exciting new area of research focussing on gut bacteria and the way it links to epigenetics is likely to offer biological future explanations for the complexities of the way in which breastfeeding protects babies from infectious and non-communicable diseases.

Breastfeeding can help mothers develop close, loving relationships

Breastfeeding is primarily a relationship that mothers have with their babies. When they hold their babies close to their bodies, and especially when they are practising skin-to-skin contact, they have surges of oxytocin and a reduction in cortisol. They are less stressed physiologically and psychologically as a result. They touch and speak more to their babies in the short and long term. Researchers have described the way mothers' and babies' bodies and brains start to work together at this time. I will discuss this important aspect more fully in Chapter 6 on mental health.

This chapter has looked at the incredible health benefits of breastfeeding for babies, mothers and society (Figure 2.1). As our main focus as community practitioners is to prevent ill health and optimise the lifelong health of the population, we need to prioritise supporting parents who wish to breastfeed.

Notes

1 Rollins, N. and Doherty, T. (2019) 'Improving breastfeeding practices at scale', *The Lancet Global Health*, 7(3), pp. e292–e293.
2 Hansen, K. (2016) 'Breastfeeding: A smart investment in people and in economies', *The Lancet*, 387(10017), p. 416.
3 UNICEF BFI, UK. (2012) 'Preventing disease and saving resources: The potential contribution of increasing breastfeeding rates in the UK'. Available at: https://discovery.dundee. ac.uk/ws/files/1290558/Preventing_disease_saving_resources.pdf
4 Pokhrel, S. *et al.* (2015) 'Potential economic impacts from improving breastfeeding rates in the UK', *Archives of Disease in Childhood*, 100(4), pp. 334–340.
5 Horta, B. L., Victora, C. G. and World Health Organization (2013) *Short-term effects of breastfeeding: a systematic review on the benefits of breastfeeding on diarrhoea and pneumonia mortality*. World Health Organization. Available at: https://apps.who.int/iris/bitstream/handle/ 10665/95585/9789241506120_eng.pdf
6 Bowatte, G. *et al.* (2015) 'Breastfeeding and childhood acute otitis media: A systematic review and meta-analysis', *Acta Paediatrica* (Oslo, Norway: 1992), 104(467), pp. 85–95.
7 Holman, R. C. *et al.* (2006) 'Necrotising enterocolitis hospitalisations among neonates in the United States', *Paediatric and Perinatal Epidemiology*, 20(6), pp. 498–506.
8 Ip, S., Chung, M., Raman, G. *et al.* (2007) *Breastfeeding and Maternal and Infant Health Outcomes in Developed Countries*. Rockville, MD: Agency for Healthcare Research and Quality.
9 Royal College of Paediatrics and Child Health (RCPCH) (2020) *State of Child Health: Insight into the State of Child Health in the UK*. Available at: https://stateofchildhealth.rcpch. ac.uk/
10 Wood, H. *et al.* (2021) 'Breastfeeding promotes early neonatal regulatory T-cell expansion and immune tolerance of non-inherited maternal antigens', *Allergy*, 76(8), pp. 2447–2460.
11 Vieira Borba, V., Sharif, K. and Shoenfeld, Y. (2017) 'Breastfeeding and autoimmunity: Programming health from the beginning', *American Journal of Reproductive Immunology*, 79, p. e12778.
12 Rito, A. I. *et al.* (2019) 'Association between characteristics at birth, breastfeeding and obesity in 22 countries: The WHO European Childhood Obesity Surveillance Initiative – COSI 2015/2017', *Obesity Facts*, 12(2), pp. 226–244.
13 Azad, M. B. *et al.* (2018) 'Infant feeding and weight gain: Separating breast milk from breastfeeding and formula from food', *Pediatrics*, 142(4), e20181092.
14 Horta, B. L., Mola, C. L. de and Victora, C. G. (2015) 'Long-term consequences of breastfeeding on cholesterol, obesity, systolic blood pressure and type 2 diabetes: A systematic review and meta-analysis', *Acta Paediatrica*, 104(S467), pp. 30–37.
15 Harder, T. *et al.* (2005) 'Duration of breastfeeding and risk of overweight: A meta-analysis', *American Journal of Epidemiology*, 162(5), pp. 397–403.
16 Arenz, S. and von Kries, R. (2005) 'Protective effect of breastfeeding against obesity in childhood', in Koletzko, B. et al. (eds) *Early Nutrition and its Later Consequences: New Opportunities*. Dordrecht: Springer Netherlands (Advances in Experimental Medicine and Biology), pp. 40–48.
17 Owen, C. G. *et al.* (2005) 'The effect of breastfeeding on mean body mass index throughout life: A quantitative review of published and unpublished observational evidence', *The American Journal of Clinical Nutrition*, 82(6), pp. 1298–1307.
18 Rito, A. I. *et al.* (2019).
19 Ibid.
20 McAndrew, F. *et al.* (2012) *Infant Feeding Survey 2010*. Available at: https://sp.ukdataservice. ac.uk/doc/7281/mrdoc/pdf/7281_ifs-uk-2010_report.pdf

21 Borra, C., Iacovou, M. and Sevilla, A. (2015) 'New evidence on breastfeeding and post-partum depression: The importance of understanding women's intentions', *Maternal and Child Health Journal*, 19(4), pp. 897–907.

22 Horta et al. (2015).

23 Su, Q. *et al.* (2021) 'Breastfeeding and the risk of childhood cancer: a systematic review and dose-response meta-analysis', *BMC Medicine*, 19(1), p. 90.

24 Silvers, K. M. *et al.* (2012) 'Breastfeeding protects against current asthma up to 6 years of age', *The Journal of Pediatrics*, 160(6), pp. 991–996.

25 Azad, M. B. *et al.* (2017) 'Breastfeeding, maternal asthma and wheezing in the first year of life: a longitudinal birth cohort study', *The European Respiratory Journal*, 49(5).

26 Hui, L. L. et al. (2019) 'Breastfeeding in infancy and lipid profile in adolescence', *Pediatrics*, 143(5), e20183075. Available at: https://publications.aap.org/pediatrics/article/143/5/e20183075/37103/Breastfeeding-in-Infancy-and-Lipid-Profile-in?autologincheck=redirected

27 Victora, C. G. *et al.* (2015) 'Association between breastfeeding and intelligence, educational attainment, and income at 30 years of age: A prospective birth cohort study from Brazil', *The Lancet Global Health*, 3(4), pp. 199–205.

28 Tambalis, K. D. *et al.* (2019) 'Exclusive breastfeeding is favorably associated with physical fitness in children', *Breastfeeding Medicine*, 14(6), pp. 390–397.

29 Aune, D. *et al.* (2014) 'Breastfeeding and the maternal risk of type 2 diabetes: A systematic review and dose-response meta-analysis of cohort studies', *Nutrition, metabolism, and cardiovascular diseases: NMCD*, 24(2), pp. 107–115.

30 Chowdhury, R. *et al.* (2015) 'Breastfeeding and maternal health outcomes: A systematic review and meta-analysis', *Acta Paediatrica* (Oslo, Norway: 1992), 104(467), pp. 96–113.

31 Chowdhury, R. *et al.* (2015) 'Breastfeeding and maternal health outcomes: A systematic review and meta-analysis', *Acta Paediatrica* (Oslo, Norway: 1992), 104(467), pp. 96–113.

32 Shenker, N. (2019) The mysteries of milk *RSB*. Available at: www.rsb.org.uk//biologist-features/158-biologist/features/1758-the-mysteries-of-milk

33 Ibid.

34 Horta, B. L. *et al.* (2013) 'Infant feeding and school attainment in five cohorts from low- and middle-income countries', *PLoS ONE*, 8(8), p. e71548.

35 Deoni, S. C. L. *et al.* (2013) 'Breastfeeding and early white matter development: A cross-sectional study', *NeuroImage*, 82, pp. 77–86.

36 Stewart, C. J. *et al.* (2018) 'Temporal development of the gut microbiome in early childhood from the TEDDY study', *Nature*, 562(7728), pp. 583–588.

37 Azad, M. B. and Kozyrskyj, A. L. (2012) 'Perinatal programming of asthma: The role of gut microbiota', *Clinical & Developmental Immunology*, 2012, p. 932072.

38 Verduci, E. *et al.* (2014) 'Epigenetic effects of human breast milk', *Nutrients*, 6(4), pp. 1711–1724

3 Why is formula feeding considered 'normal' in the UK?

How have we reached this point in time, where we as mammals are more likely to give another animal's milk to our babies rather than mothers' breastmilk?

Social attitudes have changed in the last three generations of mothers to a place where formula feeding is seen as the 'normal' way to feed babies in the UK. Many people think that formula milk, a highly processed food made from cow's milk, is similar to breastmilk and more acceptable in public places. Some families see bottle feeding with formula milk as a way to return to their pre-pregnancy lives, where feed times are more predictable, convenient and reliable. As I write this chapter, there are reports of breastmilk being artificially processed from maternal breast tissue, but the safety and efficacy of this has yet to be established. This milk will have many disadvantages when compared with mother's own milk, as it will never contain antibodies and hormones, or change as the baby grows. Several theories have been put forward suggesting how breastmilk substitutes have become an acceptable way of feeding babies. In this chapter I will include the history of infant feeding in Europe, surveys in the last 50 years, the political responses and the marketing of formula milk, plus attempts made to control its commercial promotion.

What does history tell us about infant feeding in the UK?

Complementary foods and milks in addition to breastfeeding are not unusual in history, or across the world today. During the last century, the influences of commercial companies with their clever advertising were profound. As I mentioned earlier, parents coming to the UK from countries where breastfeeding rates are high have changed their attitudes within 18 months and some who have exclusively breastfed children in their countries of origin have told me they do not have enough milk here. Some have strong cultural reasons why they want to breastfeed but find that they do not receive the support they need to do so and become 'deculturised'.[1] They have been exposed to advertising of follow-on milks and the visibility of bottle-feeding parents in public places, and some find that even healthcare professionals here may question the adequacy of mothers' breasts to nourish infants and young children. A father-to-be commented to me recently, following an online antenatal class that: 'Breastfeeding puts a lot of stress on mothers and I would like to be more involved sometimes, so could help her by giving our baby normal feeds from bottles.'

I will examine how these attitudes about infant feeding have arisen and will begin by looking at practices in Europe. Valerie Fildes,[2] in her excellent book on the history of

DOI: 10.4324/9781003139775-3

infant feeding, traces four main methods of infant feeding in Europe from 1500 to 1800. These were maternal breastfeeding, wet nursing, hand feeding and direct animal suckling.

What is the history of wet nurses, and do they exist now?

Wet nurses were often used out of necessity, following the death or illness of mothers at times when maternal and infant mortality rates were high and infectious diseases such as syphilis were common. The aristocracy or wealthy often paid for wet nurses, and this was common practice well into the last century.

These wealthy women did not breastfeed their own children as they used wet nurses, with the result that they became fertile more quickly, by missing out on the contraceptive effect of lactational amenorrhoea, so often had very large families. In pre-industrial England 18 children were not uncommon in one family and there were reports of women having up to 30 pregnancies, but many of these babies did not survive infancy.

> Not only did ordinary women breastfeed their own babies, but they suckled others, both in the day-to-day sharing of childcare and as a waged job. This protected them from the excessive fertility of noble women whose babies were wet nursed from birth.[3]

The ideal wet nurse was plump and had a good, calm, cheerful personality because there was a belief that her character was passed through her milk. They were usually highly respected in European society and were well paid. According to Palmer, foundling hospitals in London in the 18th century had a well organised wet nursing service, as it was found that a 'dry nursed' (fed another mammal's milk) baby was almost three times more likely to die than a wet nursed one. Occasionally there was some distrust in them as it was thought that they passed their characteristics through their milk.

The idea that the mother's characteristics are passed on to the baby is prevalent today in many countries and, in my research with Hindu Indian families, I was told by several mothers that they believed that the thoughts of a woman could be passed through her milk.

Islamic texts also encourage breastfeeding for 2 years and forbid marriage between people who were breastfed by the same woman because they are believed to be related to each other ('milk-kin'). Immunologists have found that cells from a mother's milk can circulate in her child's body throughout his/her life, so this belief could have some scientific backing. In Chapter 11 I will explore the impact of cultural beliefs on breastfeeding in more detail.

Many children developed close emotional relationships with their wet nurses, more than with their biological mothers, and found separating from them when weaned very difficult. Two elderly men who were born in Germany in the 1920s told me recently of the close relationships they formed with their wet nurses. One told me how he was exclusively breastfed by a 'semi-literate peasant girl' until he was 5 years old without any solid foods. After moving to a city, his mother was told by a doctor how shocked he was that her son had not been started on supplementary feeding with solids, as he had been reared entirely on breastmilk and suffered from several dietary deficiencies. He told me: 'that was what my peasant nurse thought was right and my mother was young and did not know any better.' The other man told me proudly that he was breastfed in Germany, but not by his mother!

Women still breastfeed babies other than their own in many countries around the world, for many different reasons. Perhaps the mother is not able to because she has to work, go to college, is unwell or may even have died. Sometimes it may be necessary for another woman to re-lactate to enable her to establish an adequate milk supply and even post-menopausal women can do this, especially if they have previously had a child and breastfed him/her.

I came across an interesting example of this when I was working as an infant feeding co-ordinator in a local hospital, where I met a young woman from the Middle East who had just given birth to a baby boy a few hours earlier, but he had not yet attached to her breasts. I suggested that she try to hand express some colostrum into a syringe to feed to her baby and left her with her mother, while I went to find one. When I returned, her mother, the baby's grandmother, was breastfeeding the baby! I tried not to look surprised and she told me that she was just showing her daughter and the baby what to do! She also said that she wanted to stimulate her supply, so she could feed him when her daughter returned to college. This grandmother understood how to re-lactate, through coming from a country where breastfeeding was the normal way to feed babies. These skills and knowledge have been lost in the UK today. Grandmothers here are often unable to support and give confidence to their daughters and daughters-in-law about the way babies breastfeed and how to stimulate and maintain milk supplies. I realised how far UK culture has moved away from accepting that breastfeeding may be shared with close family members and friends. However, examples of 'milk sharing' are creeping back, but these need to be done in a safe way.

Valerie Fildes explained that changes happened in Europe as suspicions started to be raised about wet nurses, especially concerns that syphilis might be transmitted to babies through their milk. This fear was unfounded, as it is transmitted through sexual contact or direct contact with sores and not through milk. As a result, in the 18th century, attempts were made to find a suitable artificial milk for babies from other mammals' milks, avoiding the use of wet nurses. These milks became popular in cooler climates in Northern Europe where animal milk was plentiful and less likely to become contaminated than in hot, humid places where they caused very high infant mortality rates. Occasionally babies were attached directly to animal teats such as sheep or goats, or this milk fed with cupped hands, but in France and Germany wet nurses continued to be used until after the Second World War, when formula feeding became safer and gained in popularity.

What have surveys in the last 50years told us about the prevalence of breastfeeding in the UK?

Infant feeding surveys have taken place every 5 years since 1975, which have not only informed us about the rates of breastfeeding over time in the UK, but also the experiences of parents and their infant feeding goals. These rich data, gathered through quantitative and qualitative methods, has also helped our understanding of women's experiences. Between 1980 and 2000 there were few changes in the initiation and continuation rates, with 67% of women in 1980, 65% in 1985, 66% in 1995 and 69% in 2000[4] starting to breastfeed after birth, followed by a rapid decline in the early weeks. There was an encouraging trend towards more UK women initiating breastfeeding with

76% in 2005 and 81% in 2010. This included all babies who were put to the breast at all, even if this was on one occasion only, and also included giving expressed breast-milk. Sadly over 72% women reported they had stopped breastfeeding before they had planned. Unfortunately, the 2015 survey was cancelled, so an accurate, recent picture of the prevalence of breastfeeding is not available, as I write, but we hope there will be a new national survey based on electronic NHS data, as well as women's experiences in 2021/22.

The highest incidences of any breastfeeding from the 2010 survey were found among:

- mothers aged 30 or over (87%),
- those from minority ethnic groups – 97% for Chinese, 96% for Black and 95% for Asian,
- those who left education aged over 18 (91%),
- those in managerial and professional occupations (90%),
- those living in the least deprived areas (89%).

While breastfeeding initiation has been steadily increasing over time, the prevalence of breastfeeding at older ages did not increase between 1995 and 2000.

The 2010 UK survey (Figure 3.1) also showed a fall from 81% at birth to 69% at one week, and 55% at 6 weeks. At 6 months, just over a third of mothers (34%) were still breastfeeding, but only 1% doing so exclusively, the lowest rate in the world.[5]

Although this initial improvement was welcome, the survey showed there was a steep drop-off in the first few weeks, due to many mothers being unable to achieve their feeding goals, leading to deep disappointment and, in some cases, anger or depression, which may become long-lasting.

The cancellation of the 2015 survey in England and the postponement of the 2020 survey because of the pandemic, means that there is no data available to inform us of the prevalence of breastfeeding, or a baseline for possible future programmes.

Public Health England now collects 'fingertips' data on breastfeeding continuation rates when babies are 6–8 weeks, but this still remains incomplete at the time of writing.[6]

Scotland carried out a survey in 2018/19, which showed improvements in initiation and continuation with almost two-thirds of babies being breastfed at birth. More than half were being breastfed at the health visitors' first postnatal visit, an increase from 44% in 2002. Improvements in rates were seen in all groups and social inequalities in breastfeeding were reducing.

How does infant feeding impact on social inequalities?

The place of residence at this time in history appears to impact on infant feeding choices, with mothers living in the most deprived areas of the UK and younger mothers shown in the surveys to be less likely to initiate and continue to breastfeed. This indicates that these babies are beginning their lives already disadvantaged in health and social terms. Sir Michael Marmot has written and broadcast widely about social inequalities in health, and parallels can be seen with breastfeeding prevalence being lower in areas of social deprivation. He previously worked with the WHO and the European Review of Social Determinants of Health and his recommendations have been adopted by the World Health Assembly and some local authorities in England.

Incidence of breastfeeding by country (1995 to 2010)

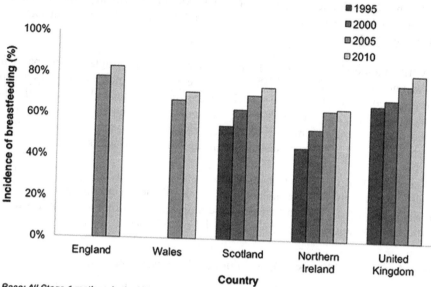

Base: All Stage 1 mothers in the UK 2010 (15724), 2005 (12290), 2000 (9492), 1995 (9130)

Figure 3.1 Infant Feeding Survey 2010
Source: McAndrew, F. *et al.* (2012). https://sp.ukdataservice.ac.uk/doc/7281/mrdoc/pdf/7281_ifs-uk-2010_report.pdf

The Fair Society Healthy Lives[7] report is very relevant to health visitors and community practitioners. It concludes that reducing health inequalities would require action on six policy objectives:

1 Give every child the best start in life.
2 Enable all children, young people and adults to maximise their capabilities and have control over their lives.
3 Create fair employment and good work for all.
4 Ensure healthy standard of living for all.
5 Create and develop healthy and sustainable places and communities.
6 Strengthen the role and impact of ill-health prevention.

Marmot argues in 'The Health Gap'[8] that there is a growing gap between social groups across the world and that health equity should be viewed as social justice. With 'proportionate universalism' there is a fairer society in which services are available to everyone. His review, published in 2020, on the social determinants of health in England, was commissioned by the Health Foundation, and shows that the gap between wealthy and deprived areas has grown since 2010. He pointed out that there are increasing numbers of children living in poverty, currently at over 30% for the UK and rising every year. He also showed that place matters and there is a gap between the deprived areas in the North and South of the country. Life expectancy for women is 5 years less in the North East of England than in similar deprived areas of London.

In addition, he has looked at the impact of Covid-19 on widening the inequalities' gap and launched *Build Back Fairer*, [9] the COVID-19 Marmot Review, in December 2020. It investigated:

> How the pandemic has affected health inequalities in England. Pre-pandemic socioeconomic and ethnic inequalities have deepened, and new inequalities are also emerging, influenced by people's work, where they live, who they live with, their ethnicity and religion. Meanwhile the impacts of containment measures on education, employment, income and local areas risk widening inequalities, including in health, in the longer term, unless urgent mitigating action is taken.

We can conclude that the Government needs to take urgent action to address the six points above and universal services should be available to all families. Increasing breastfeeding support to all families will give children and women better health outcomes and begin to address these growing social inequalities.

How has the Welfare Foods Scheme impacted breastfeeding rates?

In 1940, during the Second World War, the UK Government was concerned about the health of pregnant women and young children because milk was in short supply, so it introduced the Welfare Food Scheme. National Dried Milk, along with concentrated orange juice for vitamin C and cod liver oil for vitamins A and D, were available to all pregnant women from health visitors in well baby clinics. In the 1950s, only parents on low incomes were eligible for these welfare foods and vouchers as a nutritional safety net. In 1975 maternal and infant vitamin drops replaced the orange juice and cod liver oil and from 1977 commercial infant formula was sold in baby clinics instead of National Dried Milk.

Allowing commercial companies to sell formula milks on NHS premises gave parents the impression that these products had health service approval as a healthy way of feeding babies. One voucher could be exchanged in the clinic for a 900g tin of first stage formula (not follow-on formula milk advertised as suitable for babies over 6 months), or 7 pints of cows' milk from a supermarket. This practice continued into the late 1990s and I remember the impact this had on parents' attitudes to breastfeeding and how difficult it was for us as health visitors to support families with it, while giving out these conflicting messages in our clinics. Yes, it brought families to clinics who might not have come otherwise, but also sent out messages to communities that baby clinics promoted formula feeding. Over the 60 years while this practice continued, it contributed to shaping public attitudes away from breastfeeding.

In 2002, the Committee on Medical Aspects of Food and Nutrition[10] Policy's (COMA) Panel on Maternal and Child Nutrition published the first scientific review of the Welfare Foods Scheme since its introduction in 1940. It found that there was no incentive for mothers to breastfeed and modifications were needed. The uptake of vitamin drops was low in contrast to the high formula uptake, reflecting the low prevalence of breastfeeding. Following this report, the scheme was changed in 2004 so that vouchers could be exchanged for healthy foods and milk as well as formula milks in supermarkets, supporting the diets of pregnant women and breastfeeding mothers.

The application forms were fairly complicated to complete, not translated into other languages, apart from Welsh, and many health visitors spent a great deal of time helping families to complete them, especially those with English as a second language. The uptake of the scheme was out of reach for many families. The forms initially required signatures from midwives, health visitors or GPs, which also put barriers in the way for many parents. The aim of this scheme was to encourage families to eat more fruit and vegetables, as well as opening it up to mothers who were breastfeeding.

Unfortunately, the value of the tokens did not keep up with inflation and did not increase between 2009 and 2018. A consultation in 2018 on Healthy Start in the childhood obesity plan also considered the 2015 NICE cost-effectiveness report. The Scottish Government introduced the Best Start Foods scheme in 2018 but reported on some evidence of pregnant women stockpiling formula by exchanging their tokens, rather than buying healthy foods for themselves. Now the application forms for tokens do not have to be signed by health professionals and can be completed online. The Healthy Start Issuing Unit recommends that governments and policymakers set a target of 80% uptake for those eligible and all families have access to free pregnancy and children's vitamins.

First Steps Nutrition Trust has asked for an urgent review of the scheme, to enhance it, by including information for breastfeeding mothers on accessing support, as well as having application forms translated into other languages. This would convey a message of positive support for breastfeeding families and redress some of the messages the old Welfare Foods scheme.

Have there been national campaigns or professional positions statements to support breastfeeding?

The UK Government has launched two campaigns in the past 30 years, 'Invest in Breast Together' (1995) and 'Every Child Matters' (2003), which offered some short-term funding for breastfeeding projects, but this has not been sustained. The responsibility has been largely transferred to local public health departments, under local authorities who have found their funding to have been stretched in recent years and often breastfeeding is not seen as a high priority.

There have been some positive national statements on the importance of breastfeeding in the UK in the last 20 years by governmental agencies. In 2018, the Scientific Advisory Committee on Nutrition (SACN) issued a report on 'Feeding in the first year of life' that recommended that:

> Babies are exclusively breastfed until around 6 months of age and continue to be breastfed for at least the first year of life. Additionally, solid foods should not be introduced until around 6 months to benefit the child's overall health.[11]

This SACN report is essential reading on feeding infants and children and will both inform your practice and enable you to give parents evidence-based information.

Many of the Royal Colleges have issued position statements in the last few years, notably one published in 2017 by the Royal College of Paediatrics and Child Health (RCPCH),[12] which states that it strongly supports breastfeeding, the promotion of breastfeeding and the provision of advice and support for women, and that national policies and legislation should become conducive to breastfeeding.

The Royal College of Midwives (RCM)[13] followed with a position statement in 2018 which said that breastfeeding brings optimum health benefits to mother and baby and midwives should support all mothers who wish to do so.

The NHS Long-term Plan 2019/24 has committed to ensuring that all maternity services are working towards or have achieved UNICEF UK Baby Friendly accreditation. A financial support offer for England to aid this progress has been announced by Professor Dunkley-Bent, the Chief Midwifery Officer. The NHS Plan states that there is a commitment to:

> Improve breastfeeding rates – each maternity service will be asked to deliver an accredited, evidence-based infant feeding programme in 2019/20 – such as the UNICEF Baby Friendly initiative – which recommends exclusive breastfeeding for six months and thereafter with other foods for two years.[14]

This is very encouraging and will help hospitals achieve this award, but we hope similar support will be offered for community services to enable parents to achieve their breastfeeding goals.

What other factors influence UK public opinion today on ways of feeding babies?

Infant feeding has been an emotionally charged subject in the UK since the middle of the 20th century and often a difficult subject to raise in a social context for fear of the upset it could cause. The Government has been promoting the 'breast is best' message but has failed the mothers who had started breastfeeding and wished to continue by not providing the support they needed.

This very sad situation in which we find ourselves today in the UK can leave women with feelings of terrible guilt and loss which Amy Brown[15] (2019) describes as severe trauma that can lead to postnatal depression. She sends this message to mothers:

> You did not fail. No woman 'fails' to breastfeed. They are failed by a system that fails to support them, both during breastfeeding and when they cannot. And this is what we are going to change.

What needs to change in the UK to reverse this terrible disappointment and optimise support to new parents?

Two recent UK reports based on international standards have identified what needs to change in order to give parents the support they need to achieve their goals in infant feeding. They made recommendations to the UK Government but, to date, none of these has been implemented in the UK as a whole.

The report by the World Breastfeeding Trends Initiative (WBTi)[16] was launched in Parliament in 2016 and provided a snapshot on the state of breastfeeding in the UK. This was drawn up through a collaborative process with professional, governmental and third sector organisations to highlight successes, pinpoint gaps and map recommendations for action. The ten policy and programme and five practice indicators were assessed according to the toolkit developed by the International Baby Food Action Network (IBFAN)[17] to help countries evaluate breastfeeding policies and practices in a systematic way. They benchmark the progress in implementation of the international

Global Strategy for Infant and Young Child Feeding.[18] The indicators demonstrate how current breastfeeding policies and practices impact on breastfeeding initiation and continuation rates across the four countries of the UK. The indicators are each scored out of 10 and overall the UK scored 81.5/150. The full report and score cards can be found on the WBTi website and show that some countries score more highly than others.

The highest indicator scores were for the UNICEF UK Baby Friendly Initiative and for community-based support, notably the health visiting service (which in 2016 was better staffed than it is at the moment), but it was found that these services were often not integrated with voluntary breastfeeding support or specialist lactation services. One of the indicators which was given only a moderate score was that of health professional education. This noted that health visitor, paediatric and GP training standards/curricula contained insufficient breastfeeding components, especially on practical aspects of supporting parents to breastfeed. The steering group that drew up the report has used opportunities like consultations to try to improve pre- and post-registration training in breastfeeding.

Lowest scores were given to the stark omission of any national policy, programme and co-ordination in England and Wales. Scotland and Northern Ireland's devolved healthcare system, however, scored very highly on this indicator as it has central governmental leadership and strategies on infant feeding. The indicator on information support similarly found that there was no national, multi-media communications strategy for infant and young child feeding in England and Wales but there was in Scotland and Northern Ireland.

The lack of any national strategy for emergencies across the UK was demonstrated during the COVID-19 Pandemic, where there was no central planning for babies and new parents, adding to which many health visitors were unfortunately deployed during the first wave to work in the acute sector. Also, during this time, existing services moved away from face-to-face contacts, leaving many parents with little support, which might have long-term adverse consequences. The WBTi report of 2016 concludes with recommending that the way forward is to involve the government in formulating national strategies to drive change in a sustainable way and action is needed at every level.

A European WBTi report (2020) called 'Are our babies off to a healthy start?'[19] outlined the state of the implementation of the Global Strategy for Infant and Young Child Feeding in 18 countries. It came to a similar conclusion that the only way that change will happen is through political involvement at the highest level.

This could be achieved by countries going through the process outlined in the Becoming Breastfeeding Friendly (BBF)[20] programme, which is 'an evidence-informed global initiative designed to help countries identify the strength of their breastfeeding-friendly environment and develop recommendations as well as plans for scaling up their breastfeeding policies and programs'. The long-term objective of this initiative is to identify the concrete measures a country can take to sustainably increase its breastfeeding rates.

Some countries, notably Mexico, Brazil and Ghana, have followed this BBF model, which centres around a national strategy with political involvement, to make recommendations to government. Through this process countries have reported improvements in breastfeeding rates and in the support given to mothers. This project is led globally by Yale University. The assessment process was started in the UK in 2018, led by Kent University, who conducted research into infant feeding. The process involved Public Health England and the Scottish and Welsh devolved governments; Recommendations for change were drawn up by the working group of academics, professionals and third sector representatives for England, Wales and Scotland over a period of two years from 2017. The devolved health departments in Scotland and Wales were quick to implement these in 2019, but so far England had not done so by the middle of 2021.

A new UK Government report launched on early years

The report on Early Years (March 2021),[21] led by Andrea Leadsom MP, recommended the establishment of welcoming Family Hubs with empathy at their heart, which would replace Sure Start Centres to give families 'seamless support'. They would offer a universal service, building on an improved Start 4 life offer, including breastfeeding support. A single leader in each area would prioritise the first 1,001 critical days from conception to 2 years, offering an integrated, best practice service. There would be parents' and carers' panels to give feedback and recommendations. Political commitment to protect and support breastfeeding, together with adequate funding, is essential to ensure that parents in the future receive better support to meet their breastfeeding goals.

The recommendation on the collection of accurate national data on breastfeeding rates seems a good starting point because, at the moment, we do not know how many mothers are initiating or how long they are continuing to breastfeed. As I mentioned earlier, the last national infant feeding survey was in 2010, showing that the UK had the lowest rates of exclusive breastfeeding in the world when babies were 6 months old and many mothers reported that they did not receive the support they needed to continue to meet their breastfeeding goals. Unfortunately, as the 2015 Survey was cancelled, we have no idea whether this has improved since then, but anecdotal reports suggest that mothers are still lacking the support they would like.

How can health visitors and community practitioners improve the support given to mothers?

Health visitors are in unique key positions to begin to make these changes because we meet parents in their own homes and every new family has access to the service. We can ensure that all mothers who wish to breastfeed receive the support they ask for and can be signposted to specialist services when necessary.

For the Cochrane review in 2017 by McFadden[22] on the effectiveness of breastfeeding support, she reviewed 100 randomised controlled trials involving 83,246 women, looking at what type of support was effective and what helped them to continue to breastfeed for longer. It showed that face-to-face support was the most effective and any type of additional support was found to be helpful:

> Providing women with extra organised support helps them breastfeed their babies for longer. Breastfeeding support may be more helpful if it is predictable, scheduled, and includes ongoing visits with trained health professionals including midwives, nurses and doctors, or with trained volunteers. Different kinds of support may be needed in different geographical locations to meet the needs of the people within that location. We need additional randomised controlled studies to identify what kinds of support are the most helpful for women.

Is there such a thing as a 'free' lunch?

Have we as health visitors always given positive messages about breastfeeding? I can remember, when I was practising in the 1980s, being sent free samples of formula milks, baby rice, and dried weaning foods by companies for babies from 4 months! Also, free study days were available, (and are still being offered), sponsored by this baby feeding industry. Attending those should be considered a serious conflict of interest.

Over the decades, companies sent attractive calendars, post-its, pens, diaries etc. with names and logos on them, to midwives and health visitors, making us unpaid promoters of their formula milk products. Some things have improved but, over the past few decades, subtle messages have been given to parents (and health care professionals!) through the advertising of follow-on milks on peak-time television, online baby clubs and magazines. These include messages about the superiority of breastmilk, while at the same time making subtle comparisons to the nutritional contents of the formula products. Human milk can be absorbed easily by the baby and is a 'bioavailable' living fluid, giving lifelong health, and, as described in the last chapter, very different from this highly processed cows' milk substance. These advertisements put doubts in parents' minds about the adequacy and reliability of their supplies of breastmilk. It is no wonder that there is confusion in society! The International Code of Marketing of Breastmilk Substitutes was endorsed in 1981 by the World Health Assembly (the world's highest health policy setting body) to protect breastfeeding from aggressive marketing. The Code has been revisited in alternate years by the Assembly, resulting in subsequent Resolutions which carry equal weight to the Code. New guidance on this Code was published in 2017, where experts found that there was a lack of evidence in progress being made to eliminate harmful inappropriate marketing strategies and practices in member countries. A WHO review in 2020 of implementation of the Code by countries found that 70% of the 194 WHO Member States had enacted legal measures, with only 25 having measures substantially aligned with the Code.[23]

Governments of all four UK nations have repeatedly partially incorporated this code in law, by making it illegal to advertise first milks. However, it remains legal to advertise follow-on milks and toddler milks to the general public. These milks are considered by professionals to be unnecessary, because the first milks can be given until one year and full-fat cow's milk introduced after that, with baby vitamin supplements.

The aim of the Code is not only to protect breastfeeding, but also to ensure the proper use of breastmilk substitutes when they are required. The UN Convention on the Rights of the Child (UNCRC) also considers whether governments have implemented this Code when assessing a country. The Global Strategy for Infant and Young Child Feeding calls for all countries to implement the Code in its entirety.

Companies have found loopholes in this law to access health professionals by advertising in professional journals and providing free conferences, workshops and the health visitor of the year competitions. Perhaps practitioners feel that they can attend these and ignore any promotion of these products, but it is difficult not to pick up subliminal messages about certain products or feel grateful to the companies.

We need to remember that there is no such thing as a free lunch or free study day!

Grummer-Strawn summarises the new International Code guidance (2016 Resolution) which:

1   Clarifies that 'follow-up formula' and 'growing-up milks' that are marketed up to the age of 36 months fall under the scope of the Code and should not be promoted.
2   States that messages on complementary foods should always include a statement on the need for breastfeeding to continue through 2 years and that complementary foods should not be fed before 6 months.
3   Says that labels and designs on complementary foods need to be distinct from those used on breastmilk substitutes to avoid cross-promotion.
4   Recognizes that any donations to the health care system (including health workers and professional associations) from companies marketing BMS and foods for infants and young children represent a conflict of interest and should not be allowed.
5   Emphasizes that sponsorship of meetings of health professionals and scientific meetings by companies selling BMS and foods for infants and young children should not be allowed.[24]

Are specialist formulae necessary?

Recently, companies in the UK have been promoting milks for certain conditions such as reflux, cow's milk intolerance and colic. Although there are some babies who suffer from these conditions, they are often not diagnosed by health visitors or doctors. Instead, parents may decide spontaneously to purchase expensive, specialist formula milks from supermarkets, so are self-diagnosing. This has added to possible unnecessary anxiety and expenditure, when frequently the symptoms that babies are displaying are just those of gut immaturity, which is likely to improve with time. Reflux and regurgitation are common in many babies and keeping babies upright after feeds can often help. For bottle-fed babies, paced bottle feeding, in which the baby controls the flow and volume of milk taken, can help.

In breastfed infants, optimising effective positioning and attachment enables babies to access more of the fattier hindmilk and reduces the higher volume, higher lactose, lower calorie foremilk they can receive through poor latching.[25] This older research investigating the link between attachment of the baby's mouth and the transfer of hindmilk has often been misinterpreted. Rules have been made, wrongly about babies needing a certain length of time on the breast to access the higher calorie fattier milk. In fact, the conclusion of this research was that optimum attachment, with the baby taking a large mouthful of breast tissue with the lower lip and tongue and the mother's nipple high in the baby's mouth, was the key to effective breastfeeding.

I will describe this in more detail in Chapter 5 but would encourage all practitioners to read the insights of this work, which I will be referring to it in later chapters. It is an interesting phenomenon that society, professionals and families frequently want to make rules about breastfeeding and by doing so may misunderstand important research.

How have professional organisations responded by giving their support to the International Code of Marketing of Breastmilk Substitutes?

Some recent positive changes made by professional organisations include the Royal College of Paediatrics and Child Health stopping receiving funding from formula companies and the *British Medical Journal* and the *Community Practitioner* no longer running advertisements. The Institute of Health Visiting (iHV) and Community Practitioners' Association (CPHVA) are already Code-compliant and accept no sponsorship from formula companies. Awareness of the impact this sponsorship and advertising can have on practitioners' attitudes to infant feeding is growing, as is the need to give every family evidence-based breastfeeding support.

Why are breastfeeding mothers often hidden from the public gaze?

Breastfeeding mothers remain largely hidden from public view and are rarely portrayed on TV or seen in public places, in many parts of the UK. Many parents having their first babies have never seen a baby feeding on the breast. This is particularly the case in some areas where rates are low but, in others, such as many parts of London and the South of England, it is almost normal and acceptable to see breastfeeding mothers in cafés, supermarkets and shopping centres. Examples of celebrities breastfeeding in public places can give a positive view of the acceptability of breastfeeding away from the home. 'Brelfies' (breastfeeding selfies) have become popular images of babies breastfeeding, but sometimes the internet may place filters on such images. There are no sanctions on images of male nipples, but female ones are more likely to be hidden! It is still not widely known that the Equality Act 2010 provides a legal framework to protect the right of individuals to be free from discrimination, including breastfeeding mothers, which means they can legally breastfeed in all public places and cannot be asked to leave restaurants or cafés.

Why do women in the UK feel they need to hide their breasts in public?

Breasts have been sexualised in many industrial societies like Britain, where they can be seen in magazines as erotic images, but rarely seen for their mammalian function of feeding babies. In societies where there is no shame in breastfeeding in public places, images of breasts are not seen as sexually stimulating, but other parts of the female body may be, such as legs, face, lips and the nape of the neck. In some cultural groups, women who are not allowed to show their faces in public can show their breasts when feeding babies. I will be discussing different cultural beliefs around breastfeeding in Chapter 11.

Can parents access good support online?

Social media can be an amazing support for mothers if they have access to the internet and can access reliable, trustworthy sources of information, but can also be a source of confusion when information is not evidence-based. Formula companies also have sites and baby clubs which may appear to give advice on breastfeeding but may direct unsuspecting parents to their products. Although face-to-face contact with trained health professionals, counsellors or peer supporters are mothers' preferred ways of getting help, there were examples during the COVID-19 pandemic in many areas of health visitors setting up effective online support. There are local and national Facebook groups which have become virtual communities where breastfeeding parents can find support at any time which is convenient for them, and I have heard of many mothers who connect with each other in the middle of the night!

An online survey of 2,028 mothers revealed that local breastfeeding Facebook groups are very common across the UK today and, on this platform, parents are able to connect with peer supporters and other mothers enabling immediate, daily contact. They reported how much they valued the convenience of this support and many kept in contact with the group until their children reached toddlerhood.[26]

How can community practitioners influence societal change?

There are ways that we can influence change in our local communities. We can call on shops and restaurants to be breastfeeding-friendly and ensure that our own workplaces support breastfeeding staff returning to work, by providing areas where they can express their milk or breastfeed their babies. We need to avoid this sad situation where I was told by a midwife that she had to breastfeed her baby in her car, when her partner brought her baby to the hospital where she worked to feed in the middle of her shift.

What we really need to address is the fact that the UK's low breastfeeding rates are a serious public health issue. We need to ensure we have breastfeeding training to support families with evidence-based information and uphold the International Code of marketing breastmilk substitutes, to ensure that we are not promoting formula milks as superior or equivalent to breastmilk in any way. We also need to address the barriers that stop women breastfeeding in our local communities and support them to follow their chosen method of feeding, thus meeting their goals and avoiding the upset and grief of not achieving them. We can put pressure on our local and national governments to show leadership and respond to the overwhelming evidence around the benefits of breastfeeding.

In the next chapter we will look at how we can understand our own attitudes and communicate effectively. Through listening to parents, using counselling skills and providing evidence-based practical support, we can help them achieve their infant feeding goals.

Notes

1 Hutton, E. and Raven, J. (2016) 'Exploring the infant feeding practices of immigrant women in the North West of England: A case study of asylum seekers and refugees in Liverpool and Manchester', *Maternal & Child Nutrition*, 12(2), pp. 299–313.
2 Fildes, V. A. (1986) *Breasts, Bottles and Babies: A History of Infant Feeding*. Edinburgh: Edinburgh University Press.
3 Palmer, G. (2009, 2011) *The Politics of Breastfeeding: When Breasts are Bad for Business*. London: Pinter & Martin.
4 Hamlyn, B. and UK Statistics Authority (2002) *Infant feeding 2000: A survey conducted on behalf of the Department of Health, the Scottish Executive, the National Assembly for Wales and the Department of Health, Social Services and Public Safety in Northern Ireland*. London: TSO.
5 McAndrew, F. *et al.* (2012) *Infant Feeding Survey 2010*. Available at: https://sp.ukdataservice.ac.uk/doc/7281/mrdoc/pdf/7281_ifs-uk-2010_report.pdf
6 Public Health England (PHE) (2021) *Child and Maternal Health*. Available at: https://fingertips.phe.org.uk/profile/child-health-profiles/data
7 The Health Foundation (2020) *Health Equity in England: The Marmot Review 10 Years On*. Available at: www.health.org.uk/publications/reports/the-marmot-review-10-years-on
8 Marmot, M. (2017) 'The health gap: The challenge of an unequal world: the argument', *International Journal of Epidemiology*, 46(4), pp. 1312–1318.
9 The Health Foundation (2020) *Build Back Fairer: The COVID-19 Marmot Review*. Available at: www.health.org.uk/publications/build-back-fairer-the-covid-19-marmot-review
10 Gov.UK (2002) *Scientific Review of the Welfare Food Scheme*. Available at: https://assets.publishing.service.gov.uk/government/uploads/system/uploads/attachment_data/file/743512/Scientific_Review_of_the_Welfare_Food_Scheme__2002_

11 Gov.UK (2017) *Feeding in the First Year of Life: SACN Report*. Available at: www.gov.uk/government/publications/feeding-in-the-first-year-of-life-sacn-report

12 Royal College of Paediatrics and Child Health (RCPCH) (2017) *Breastfeeding in the UK – Position Statement*. Available at: www.rcpch.ac.uk/resources/breastfeeding-uk-position-statement

13 Royal College of Midwives (RCM) (2018) *New Position Statement on Infant Feeding*. Available at: www.rcm.org.uk/news-views/news/rcm-publishes-new-position-statement-on-infant-feeding/

14 NHS England (2019) *Long-Term Plan*. Available at: www.longtermplan.nhs.uk

15 Brown, A. (2019) *Why Breastfeeding Grief and Trauma Matter*. London: Pinter & Martin.

16 WBTi (2016) *Breastfeeding Trends (UK)*. Available at: https://ukbreastfeeding.org/about/www.worldbreastfeedingtrends.org/uploads/resources/document/wbti-tool-2019.pdf

17 Gupta, A. *et al.* (2019) 'The world breastfeeding trends initiative: Implementation of the global strategy for infant and young child feeding in 84 countries', *Journal of Public Health Policy*, 40(1), pp. 35–65.

18 WHO (2020) *Global Strategy for Infant and Young Child Feeding*. Available at: www.who.int/nutrition/publications/infantfeeding/9241562218/en/

19 Zakarija-Grković, I. *et al.* (2020) 'Are our babies off to a healthy start? The state of implementation of the global strategy for infant and young child feeding in Europe', *International Breastfeeding Journal*, 15(1), p. 51.

20 Yale School of Public Health (2017) *Becoming Breastfeeding Friendly: A Guide to Global Scale Up*. Available at: https://publichealth.yale.edu/bfci/

21 Gov.UK (2021) *The Best Start for Life: A Vision for the 1,001 Critical Days*. Available at: www.gov.uk/government/publications/the-best-start-for-life-a-vision-for-the-1001-critical-days

22 McFadden, A. *et al.* (2017) 'Support for healthy breastfeeding mothers with healthy term babies', *Cochrane Database of Systematic Reviews*. Edited by Cochrane Pregnancy and Childbirth Group.

23 UNICEF (2020) *Marketing of Breast-Milk Substitutes: National Implementation of the International Code*. Available at: www.unicef.org/reports/marketing-of-breast-milk-substitutes-status-report-2020

24 Grummer-Strawn, L. M. *et al.* (2017) 'New World Health Organization guidance helps protect breastfeeding as a human right', *Maternal & Child Nutrition*, 13(4), p. e12491.

25 Woolridge, M. W. and Fisher, C. (1988) 'Colic, "overfeeding", and symptoms of lactose malabsorption in the breast-fed baby: A possible artifact of feed management?', *The Lancet*, 332(8607), pp. 382–384.

26 Morse, H. and Brown, A. (2021) 'Accessing local support online: Mothers' experiences of local Breastfeeding Support Facebook groups', *Maternal & Child Nutrition*, 17(4), e13227.

4 Communication skills, emotional support and motivational interviewing

As I discussed in the last chapter, many women in the UK stop breastfeeding before they wish and, in the 2010 survey, only 1% were doing it exclusively at 6 months, the lowest rate in the world! We have a very unhappy situation where many women are not able to meet their infant feeding goals and some feel that they have failed their babies. This can impact on mothers' relationships with their infants and may lead to poor mental health outcomes for themselves. In this chapter, I will explore how health visitors can support parents to achieve their goals, by becoming aware of their own attitudes and through using non-directive, person-centred counselling skills and motivational interviewing techniques.

We need to change the conversation about breastfeeding in the UK

We have a dilemma in the UK when talking about breastfeeding as it runs the risk of upsetting parents and grandmothers, who may have wanted to do so, but felt they had to stop before they wished, through lack of support from professionals, families or society at large.

Sue Ashmore, Programme Director of Unicef UK Baby Friendly Initiative, called for a change of conversation in 2016 in her blog:

> We need to change the conversation. We can stop laying the blame for a major public health issue in the laps of individual women and acknowledge the collective responsibility of us all to remove the barriers to breastfeeding which lead to eight out of 10 women reporting they had to stop breastfeeding before they had wanted to.[1]

Sue Ashmore also wrote in the Community Practitioner in 2017:

> Last year, we launched a campaign to 'Change the conversation' around breastfeeding. We wanted to stop the pressure piled onto individual women to breastfeed, and instead build an environment that is supportive of women, by removing the barriers that block successful breastfeeding.[2]

In our 'Change the conversation' campaign, we're calling on health departments across England, Northern Ireland, Scotland and Wales to lead the way in removing the barriers to breastfeeding. These are many and varied, and include:

DOI: 10.4324/9781003139775-4

- Insufficient professional support to get breastfeeding off to a good start
- Not enough community support to deal with problems a bit further down the line
- A lack of understanding about how important breastfeeding is for health and brain development.[3]

The way we communicate with women and families is vital, as this needs to be done sensitively if we are to avoid the hurt they may be feeling at the moment. All new parents want to do the best they can for their children. We know that over 80% start breastfeeding but find that they lack both the internal confidence and the external support from professionals, families and society to continue for as long as they planned. Any amount of breastmilk is valuable to their babies, and even a few drops of colostrum can help babies' immunity and should be valued. Exclusive breastfeeding will give the optimum protection against diseases, as explained in Chapter 2, but for many women in the UK this is just not attainable because of lack of support, societal attitudes and beliefs, rather than a physiological inability to make enough milk.

Women who are white British and living in socio-economically deprived areas, as well as young mothers, are at higher risk of stopping before they wish to. All the surveys since 1975 have shown a geographical difference, with London having the highest prevalence of breastfeeding and the North of England, Scotland and Northern Ireland having lower rates. Social and health inequalities are growing in the UK, and not breastfeeding adds to this imbalance, with babies beginning their lives with disadvantages. Women in BAME groups are more likely to begin breastfeeding but may find it more difficult to access support outside their families. The COVID-19 pandemic appears to have accentuated this unequal situation. Additional targeted peer support programmes could help support women in your caseload you have identified as less likely to breastfeed.

As I mentioned earlier, in recent years the devolved governments of Scotland, Wales and Northern Ireland have put more resources into supporting women in an attempt to rectify this, but England has not yet done so, at the time of writing. As health visitors, we have a responsibility to listen to women to establish what their infant feeding goals are and signpost them to appropriate support.

Why understanding our own, personal attitudes is important when supporting parents

We all come into the profession with our own attitudes, which have been moulded by our personal upbringing, family and training experiences of breastfeeding. If you have been lucky enough to be able to talk about these with others and explore them in a systematic way, you may have been able to come to terms with them, and leave them in the back of your mind, so they do not invade your thoughts when listening to parents. If you are a student reading this, it is worth asking your tutors if they could facilitate you to do this.

If this is not possible, you could talk to a friend or colleague and draw your own 'time-line' of your personal experiences of infant feeding, starting off from when you were born and if you and your siblings were breastfed. Then you work through your childhood, teenage years and adult life, writing down what you remember hearing about or seeing women breastfeeding, and which people may have had an impact on how you feel about it. If you are happy sharing this with a friend, it may help you reflect on your attitudes. Once you realise that it may be unhelpful to share your own personal experiences of infant feeding with your clients, and that everyone's situation is different, you will be more open to listening to them and enabling them to formulate their own plans, build confidence and self-efficacy. It may be worth reflecting now on how you would feel if you had a problem you wanted to solve and started talking about this with friends. I would guess that the last thing you want them to do is to tell you that they had a similar problem and how they resolved it without listening to your story.

We are all members of a society which has problems accepting that breastfeeding is a reliable way of feeding babies. Surveys in the UK, since the 1970s, have shown that mothers worry about making enough milk for their babies. Understandably, some families may want to protect new mothers from these concerns by suggesting they give formula bottles as the solution. I discussed in the last chapter how the historical and political influences may have influenced societal beliefs, along with advertisements aimed at parents and health professionals. Even though we may think we are not affected by these and our practise is guided by the science and the evidence base, the subliminal messages we receive will have an impact. Awareness of these and exploring our own experiences can help us be more open to hearing what parents are actually saying to us. The reality is that many women in the UK stop breastfeeding before they wish to but many of them could carry on with appropriate support.

How can health visitors support families to build their confidence and self-efficacy to breastfeed?

Communicating with expectant and new parents requires an open, non-judgemental approach, where listening to their feelings and infant feeding goals and expectations is paramount. As health visitors, we have unique opportunities at our mandated contacts to use open questions, which can encourage parents to clarify their thoughts on the subject. I will explore these non-directive, person-centred counselling skills, which will enable you to do this effectively and empathise with their individual situations. There is some evidence that this approach is an effective way of supporting parents.

Alison McFadden's systematic review and meta-analysis of the use of 'counselling' skills for breastfeeding support looked at the evidence for effectiveness. She considered data from 26 countries across the world, ranging from high to low-income ones,[4] and used the WHO definition of breastfeeding counselling:

> The World Health Organization defines breastfeeding counselling as the support of mothers and infants, as provided by healthcare workers, in decision-making, overcoming difficulties, and implementation of optimal feeding practices … A key element is the interaction that takes places between a healthcare worker and mother, which should support women and their decision-making. Counselling is therefore a type of preventative intervention which places emphasis on the dyadic interaction between a healthcare worker and a mother, rather than the top-down approach often more characteristic of education-based types of interventions. Counselling is therefore a type of support delivered directly to mothers and infants. All counselling can be considered support but not all support interventions involve counselling.

The meaning of 'counselling' varied in several countries and was not always the full humanistic approach advocated by Carl Rogers, as we know it in the UK.

She found that when health professionals used this approach, rather than trying to problem-solve and offer advice, they were more effective. Through listening to parents and supporting them in building confidence to find their own solutions, they were more likely to meet their infant feeding goals and breastfeed for longer. This counselling support can be offered face-to-face, on the telephone, both antenatally and postnatally, and offered to all expectant parents and those with young children. She concluded that this breastfeeding counselling approach is an effective public health intervention, to increase rates of any and exclusive breastfeeding in all countries.

If this counselling approach is used by all who support parents, it can help them become confident in their skills, recognise their babies' responses, cues and needs for comfort through feeding, improve their understanding of breastfeeding and signs that adequate milk is being transferred. Counselling in this situation refers to using some of the following person-centred approaches which will help you understand the parents' lived experience.

What are the principles of person-centred communication skills?

Active listening

Listening to parents' stories can be very interesting and revealing and tells you how they feel about feeding their babies. You could ask some open questions, such as those beginning with 'what', 'how' or 'could you tell me about …' to encourage exploration of their journeys from the births of their babies and how they felt about them, which will enable them to delve into any challenging areas. When possible, it is helpful to include fathers or partners in this contact because their support and confidence in breastfeeding is essential if mothers are going to build confidence and self-efficacy. They can be there with them on those difficult days, which all parents experience, and recognise signs that their babies are breastfeeding well to reassure them, or if not, where they can help them find support.

Reflecting and clarifying

After listening to parents, you can reflect back to them some of the words or themes they are saying to you, by either parroting back their actual words, or summarising what you have been told. If you get this right, they will realise that you have heard and understood what they have been saying. If you do not get it completely correct, they will come back to you with what they really said, which in turn will help them clarify their own thoughts and will show them that you have been listening.

Being non-judgemental

It is important that you do not judge them, because they are likely to have acted in what they thought was the best way with the information they had at the time. When they express ideas with which you do not agree, you can work with them exploring ways to make changes, so they can come to their own conclusions. A non-judgemental approach that is sensitive to the parents' feelings and attitudes is essential to build their confidence and self-reliance in caring for their children. It may be helpful to practise this approach with colleagues and friends and you will be amazed how much difference it makes.

A recent (2020) survey and qualitative interviews involving half a million parents across the UK, was carried out by the Royal Foundation to ascertain the impact that COVID-19 has had on their feelings as parents, their mental health and how this impacted on their children's brain development. The Duchess of Cambridge spoke of how families were struggling during the pandemic.[5] One shocking finding was that 70% of parents were feeling judged by others, by families, society and health professionals, and sadly this led to them feeling uncomfortable about asking for help. This was most marked in parents living in socially disadvantaged areas of the UK.

Empathy

Health visitors who are empathic to parents' concerns, meaning they see the concerns from the parents' point of view, are less likely to be directive and give quick solutions, but to work with them to find the course of action they wish to take. If you can try to understand their situations and imagine yourself in their shoes this will help. It may be that mothers feel they have explored all avenues to overcome their breastfeeding challenges, but none of them seem to be helping. Also, it may be impacting on their relationship with their babies and their own mental health. They may make the decision to introduce a supplementary feed of formula in addition to breastfeeding and look for affirmation from you to do this and not feel judged. Mothers' mental health will impact on their relationships with their babies and in turn infant mental health. I will be discussing this important subject in Chapter 7.

Giving information

You can give them appropriate information on the practicalities of breastfeeding such as the importance of the signs of optimum positioning and attachment, and how to practise responsive feeding, which I will discuss in the next chapter. Try when possible to listen to their requests for information and not over-burden them with lots of facts. Many parents are confused by the conflicting information they see on the Internet and may ask for your help in sorting out what is helpful and evidence based. Some parents may decide that partial breastfeeding is their goal and ask for your support with this. Although we saw in the previous chapter that exclusive breastfeeding confers the best health outcomes, mixed feeding will still give babies some health benefits. By listening to their wishes, you will enable them to decide the direction they wish to follow, rather than give them directive advice.

Your role is to build both parents' confidence in breastfeeding, either exclusive or partial, and signpost ways in which they can find peer or specialist support when needed.

What does other research tell us about effective support?

I will now examine some of the qualitative research which looks at effective support that adds to our understanding of how women perceive effective support.

Pat Hoddinott, a GP and breastfeeding researcher in Scotland[6] led a study finding out the reactions of 36 women and 26 partners to health professionals' support. She found that there were *pivotal points* when women were more likely to give up breastfeeding and identified the immediate postnatal period after birth as a time to have realistic discussions, with *proactive* care being more effective than *reactive*.

She found that women/family-centred communication with open questions, focussing on their emotional issues, and sitting with them during a feed, helped to build their confidence. She recommended that we need to move away from breastfeeding being seen as an individual act to being situated in a wider family and social context. I find the following quote from Pat Hoddinott in which a woman decided to mix feed her baby but did not feel judged by her health visitor, very insightful:

Woman: 'That first weekend we gave him a bottle. "That's fine ... we call that a crisis bottle," she [health visitor] went, "and there's nothing wrong with that. If it works for you, that's fine" so if anything she was a bit more encouraging'. (Interview in 2003, 3 weeks after birth: breastfeeding, with formula introduced at 1 week)

Woman: 'I think if it hadn't been for that explanation [from the health visitor], I may well have sort of said, "well I've tried my best, I'm giving up." So I'm glad I didn't, and I didn't because of the health visitor, because she was so reassuring.'

The conclusions of this study were that effective, proactive support that identified achievable goals using a family-centred approach, through looking at a feeding continuum, would be more effective and more likely to lead to behavioural change than a cognitive model which focusses on the pros and cons.

This approach need not take extra time, and I know how we are all under work time pressures. A proactive approach that identifies any potential problems before they arise has been shown to be more effective. You could observe a full breastfeed while you carry out the new baby contact, if you arrange it in advance, so that the mother knows you would like to observe her breastfeeding while you are there with her at home. The other discussions you need to have with her can take place while she is feeding. You can signpost her to local breastfeeding support groups or specialist support if she needs them.

Another qualitative study[7] by Gill Thomson looked at the lack of perceived social support and how this influences women's feeding behaviour by using an 'infant feeding genogram'. This involved the parents drawing up a simple family tree before the birth of the baby, and identifying which members would be supportive of them with breastfeeding, rather than those who might have more negative attitudes. This is a way for women to map and explore their social landscape of infant feeding. The women in the study were able to draw and visualise 'asset-based' infant feeding help from their families and communities. This study was undertaken in areas of low breastfeeding rates in the UK and interviewed 103 women and analysed 32 genograms. The conclusion was that the genogram has the potential to enable women and families to identify for themselves their family and community-centred support for breastfeeding. This method could be a useful exercise for parents at your antenatal or new baby contacts.

An important meta-synthesis was carried out by Schmeid examining the evidence of 31 qualitative studies and some large surveys which focussed on formal professional and peer breastfeeding support.[8] The researcher identified a continuum from 'authentic presence' at one end, from a person who could give a mother effective support with breastfeeding to 'disconnected encounters' at the other end, which were ineffective, discouraging or counterproductive. She examined the efficacy of both peer and professional support by examining women's perceptions of their experiences and concluded that continuity of caregiver, whether professional or peer supporter, would be more likely to facilitate an 'authentic presence', especially where supportive care and a trusting relationship had been formed.

The findings of these three qualitative studies were that mother-centred, non-directive use of communication skills with open questions helped to build trusting relationships between parents and professionals or peer supporters, which enabled mothers to gain confidence and self-efficacy in their abilities to breastfeed.

Motivational interviewing techniques use this approach and have been shown to be very effective.[9]

The focus here is on behaviour change, so it is not entirely non-directive, but uses some person-centred approaches through four key processes:

- Engaging and building a trusting relationship with clear mutually agreed goals
- Evoking the client's motivation for change
- Clarifying the direction of change
- Planning how change will happen.

Techniques employed to achieve these are person-centred counselling skills:

- Asking open questions
- Actively listening with reflections
- Affirming the mother's strengths and abilities
- Summarising in your own words what you have heard
- Offering information when requested by the mother to build on her knowledge and skills
- Building her confidence
- Enabling her to identify her social support network
- Signposting to peer or specialist support when appropriate.

A novel motivational interviewing programme called 'Mam-Kind' was carried out by informed breastfeeding peer supporters to support women with breastfeeding in areas of the UK with low breastfeeding rates. A peer supporter had at least one antenatal contact with the expectant woman and another soon after the birth, with the intention to provide affirmation and signpost mothers to other sources of support, such as groups or online communities. Mothers identified areas that needed to change in order to breastfeed for longer. These peer supporters worked by building mothers' knowledge and skills and boosting their confidence through social support. The peer supporters needed certain qualities to do this work, which were that they were supportive, positive, non-judgemental, approachable, honest, down-to-earth and good listeners. They worked closely with midwives and health visitors and referred any more complex problems to them.

How can we communicate with and support fathers and partners?

The interventions above are directed at mothers, but there is a growing awareness that the support of partners is key to their confidence. A systematic review exploring fathers' views was carried out by Sharon Baldwin[10] but many of the findings could be applied to same sex or trans-gender partners. The study looked at first-time fathers' experiences of their transition to parenthood and included 351 qualitative studies between 1960 and 2017 covering many countries.

The findings of this study were revealing as they outlined the challenges fathers faced and how this can impact on their future mental health. Some fathers struggled with their transition to their new identity and changes in their relationship (especially sexual) with their partner. Many suggested that better preparation before their babies were born would help them adjust to their new role and benefit their mental well-being. Fathers and partners face competing areas of their lives such as the balance between work demands and time spent with their children.

Breastfeeding appeared to be a difficult challenge for many fathers as it was very time-consuming for mothers and they often felt pushed out. Their lifestyles had changed, which led to feelings of stress and escape activities such as smoking, working longer hours or listening to music. Fathers said that wanted more guidance and support around their preparation for fatherhood and how their relationships with partners will change. They found that barriers to accessing support were the lack of tailored information resources, and acknowledgement from health professionals of their vital role.

We can see from this research how very important it is to include fathers and partners in antenatal groups or face-to-face discussions, exploring how they can be involved in caring for their babies and bonding with them. Health visitors and midwives have opportunities to communicate effectively with them at antenatal and postnatal visits. Baldwin concluded her study by summarising the challenges facing fathers when their partners were breastfeeding:

> Men experienced a number of competing demands as they became fathers. They had to balance work demands with the time they were able to spend with their child. They also experienced a deterioration in their relationship with their partner, which included reduced satisfaction with their sexual relationship. Expectations of new fathers often did not meet reality, especially around breastfeeding and bonding. New fathers found breastfeeding to be a more difficult experience than anticipated, while many also struggled to bond with their babies in utero and in the early days following birth.

Another recent study carried out by Crippa in Italy on 300 fathers explored fathers' knowledge and overall attitude toward breastfeeding and emphasised the importance of including fathers in the promotion of breastfeeding. It was suggested that the classic mother–baby dyad could be expanded to a more modern 'mother–father–baby triad' which may improve breastfeeding outcomes at discharge from hospital.[11]

If we can engage with fathers or partners at the antenatal contact, we can discuss the realities of breastfeeding and how vital their support is. By introducing this idea of a 'breastfeeding triad', they can begin to understand that, without their support, mothers may find breastfeeding very hard, if not impossible.

How can breastfeeding peer supporters complement the support given by healthcare staff?

Throughout history women have sought support with breastfeeding from other more experienced mothers in their communities in towns and villages. The embodied knowledge of the skills required have been lost in the last three generations in Western societies and when women do not realise that breastfeeding does not come to them instinctively, they turn to professional or lay support. Peer supporters can communicate with women at an equal level, because they have had recent lived experience of breastfeeding. They carry no power imbalance or authority and mothers may talk to them more openly about sensitive, emotional issues that they may not want to share with healthcare professionals.

Peer support began in the 1950s in the USA. La Leche League (LLL) mothers began to meet in their houses to support each other with experience-based breastfeeding, because doctors they saw had little knowledge on the practicalities and emotions associated with breastfeeding and midwives did not exist. The book *The Womanly Art of Breastfeeding* was published and is still available.[12]

Following on from this, in the 1960s–70s in the UK, third sector organisations, the National Childbirth Trust (NCT) and La Leche League Great Britain (LLLGB) started training mothers who had personal breastfeeding experience to become breastfeeding counsellors. La Leche Leaders, supporting mothers in a non-directive, non-medicalised way, but with evidence-based knowledge of practical and emotional issues associated with breastfeeding. The NCT initially trained 'breastfeeding friends', who were women who had breastfed their own children but some decided to follow the more extensive training required to qualify as a breastfeeding counsellor. Later, in 1979 and 1997 respectively, the Association of Breastfeeding Mothers (ABM) and the Breastfeeding Network (BfN) were set up by existing breastfeeding counsellors and also started training mothers with personal experience of breastfeeding.

Breastfeeding peer supporters naturally followed on from these, but did not receive the extensive training of breastfeeding counsellors following the LLL model.

Peer supporters complete a training programme in practical breastfeeding and how to use mother-centred communication skills. These training programmes are often run by one of the third sector breastfeeding organisations, but sometimes local areas run their own 'in-house' training programmes. In many areas in the UK today, they are an integral part of the infant feeding team either in a paid or volunteer capacity in communities and hospitals. Unfortunately, with the economic squeeze in public health of recent years, many of these services have been cut and funding withdrawn, despite the cost-saving argument, which would result in enabling more women to breastfeed their babies.

They can complement the work of health visitors and midwives by working with the infant feeding leads, helping to run support groups in the community and possibly working in hospitals on postnatal wards in paid or volunteer roles. They can relate to women because they have similar characteristics in many ways, such as in age, ethnicity, social group and living in the locality. Through their own experiences they can empathise with any challenges or difficulties the mothers may be having. As they usually live locally, they have knowledge of local facilities such as children's centres and mothers' groups and can meet parents informally in cafés and parks. Most of them have young children and are able to relate and empathise with new parents.

While I was infant feeding lead in the community, I worked with an amazing group of breastfeeding peer supporters from different ethnic communities, speaking over 20 different languages between them, representing our local community profile. They understood cultural beliefs and practices, which made it easier for them to communicate and empathise with mothers from their groups. Some worked as volunteers or in paid positions in the local hospital and others ran targeted groups in the community. Others helped to run breastfeeding drop-in support groups and often kept in touch with mothers between group sessions by telephone, when mothers requested more support. Extra targeted support was given to women who were less likely to breastfeed, such as young mothers, those expecting or breastfeeding twins and certain ethnic groups.

Peer supporters met mothers from these groups in the antenatal period and then supported them after their babies were born. Over a period of five years, breastfeeding began to be 'normalised' in the community and it was noticed that mothers felt happier to feed their babies in public places. Health visitors and midwives all received the Unicef Baby Friendly training and worked closely with these peer supporters, recognising that they complemented their work and referred mothers directly for their support. Many mothers find breastfeeding difficult, lacking support from family and friends not only for practical reasons, which will be addressed in the next chapter, but find they also have emotional and social difficulties which they may wish to share with others.

How has the COVID-19 pandemic affected the way community practitioners communicated with families?

The pandemic has presented difficulties for pregnant and new mothers, as many not only feel isolated from family and friends, but communication with health professionals in many cases has been online. The Babies in Lockdown Report reported on a survey of 5,000 parents carried out in 2020 by three charities supporting parents – Best Beginnings, Home Start and Parent–Infant Foundation. Its aim was to investigate the impact of the pandemic on families. It found that COVID-19 affected parents, babies and services in different ways and those families at risk of poor outcomes suffered the most. Black, Asian and ethnic minority groups were hit the hardest, so widening health inequalities. Parents reported being more anxious, and having problems accessing mental health support and professional support with caring for their children. It concluded that the pandemic will cast a long shadow, with increased stresses continuing for years to come. The charities called for a 'baby boost' funding for families who had babies born during lockdown, a new 'Parent–Infant Premium' and sustained investment in support for families, with more parental involvement in planning services.

How did some charities and health visiting services continue to communicate with families through online platforms?

Where face-to-face contact was not possible, some health visitors and voluntary support services adapted quickly to offer online breastfeeding support to families. Some very successful, virtual, free antenatal information and postnatal breastfeeding support groups were set up during the first wave of the pandemic, such as Blossom Antenatal, as classes and groups were cancelled.[13] Although communication was more challenging, it enabled many parents to feel supported if they had access to the Internet. Families who did not have Internet access were seriously disadvantaged at this time, which is likely to lead to an increase in health inequalities.

The National Breastfeeding Helpline[14] spoke to a record number of parents, offering them support using counselling skills. The other breastfeeding charities also reported record numbers of calls from isolated parents asking for support and many downloaded and used the excellent, free Baby Buddy App,[15] which gave them easy access to evidence-based information.

Health visitors in many areas set up comprehensive breastfeeding support services during the pandemic, through novel ways showing courage, as they planned to communicate with families online in an innovative way. A very successful example of this was reported in the IHV publication 'Making History – Health Visiting during COVID-19'.[16] Here, four NHS trusts in Devon came together to support families. Staff trained rapidly in setting up video teleconferencing support and accessed training on how to assess infant feeding remotely. They were given opportunities to ask questions and receive support and supervision from the team, consisting of infant feeding leads, specialists and peers. The aim was to offer parents consistent messages and keep the family and child in focus at all times. A 'virtual latch' group session was set up for mothers who were struggling with this. Parents reported a high degree of satisfaction with this service at such a difficult time, when normal services were suspended. Although communication was not as easy as face-to-face, the parents felt supported and could access support easily.

In this chapter, I have outlined some of the communication skills which you are likely to find will help you communicate and support breastfeeding families in your caseload. I have also looked at some of the research evidence behind a non-directive approach, whether face-to-face or online. It will be important in your practice that you access ongoing training, professional support and supervision on communication skills, to work effectively with families.

Notes

1 Ashmore, S. (2016) 'Changing the conversation around breastfeeding', Unicef UK Baby Friendly Initiative. Available at: www.unicef.org.uk/babyfriendly/changing-conversation-around-breastfeeding

2 Ashmore, S. (2017) 'Breastfeeding: Breaking down barriers' *Community Practitioner*. Available at: www.communitypractitioner.co.uk/opinion/2017/03/breastfeeding-breaking-down-barriers

3 Ibid.

4 McFadden, A. *et al.* (2019) 'Counselling interventions to enable women to initiate and continue breastfeeding: A systematic review and meta-analysis', *International Breastfeeding Journal*, 14(1), p. 42.

5 Royal Foundation (2020) 'The Duchess of Cambridge and the Royal Foundation release the #5BigInsights in the biggest ever study on the early years'. Available at: https://royalfoundation.com/the-duchess-of-cambridge-unveils-five-big-insights-research-early-years/

6 Hoddinott, P. *et al.* (2012) 'A serial qualitative interview study of infant feeding experiences: Idealism meets realism', *BMJ Open*, 2(2), p. e000504.

7 Thomson, G. *et al.* (2020) 'Exploring the use and experience of an infant feeding genogram to facilitate an assets-based approach to support infant feeding', *BMC Pregnancy and Childbirth*, 20(1), p. 569.

8 Schmied, V. *et al.* (2011) 'Women's perceptions and experiences of breastfeeding support: A metasynthesis', *Birth*, 38(1), pp. 49–60.

9 Phillips, R. *et al.* (2018) 'Development of a novel motivational interviewing (MI) informed peer-support intervention to support mothers to breastfeed for longer', *BMC Pregnancy and Childbirth*, 18(1), p. 90.

10 Baldwin, S. *et al.* (2018) 'Mental health and wellbeing during the transition to fatherhood: A systematic review of first time fathers' experiences', *JBI Database of Systematic Reviews and Implementation Reports*, 16(11), pp. 2118–2191.

11 Crippa, B. L. *et al.* (2021) 'From dyad to triad: a survey on fathers' knowledge and attitudes toward breastfeeding', *European Journal of Pediatrics*, 180, pp. 2861–2869.

12 Weissinger, D., West, D. and Pitman, T. (2010) *The Womanly Art of Breastfeeding*. Oxford: Blackwells. Available at: https://blackwells.co.uk/bookshop/product/The-Womanly-Art-of-

Breastfeeding-by-Diane-Wiessinger-Diana-West-Teresa-Pitman-La-Leche-League-International/9781905177400

13 Blossom (2020). *Antenatal Breastfeeding Class.* Available at: www.blossomantenatal.com/breastfeeding-class

14 Breastfeeding Helplines (2021) *The Breastfeeding Network.* Available at: www.breastfeedingnetwork.org.uk/contact-us/helplines/

15 Best Beginnings (2021) 'Baby Buddy App'. Available at: www.bestbeginnings.org.uk/baby-buddy

16 IHV (2020) 'Health visiting making history: Case studies'. Available at: https://ihv.org.uk/wp-content/uploads/2021/07/Health-visiting-making-history-case-studies-FINAL-VERSION-updated-14.7.21.pdf

5 The practical skills which should help community practitioners to support parents with breastfeeding

This chapter will look at the practical information and skills which will help you support parents with breastfeeding at different stages of their babies' lives. The importance of proper attachment and positioning only began to be appreciated over 30 years ago by Chloe Fisher, a midwife in Oxford. Unfortunately, many parents, families and healthcare professionals have lost the knowledge and skills of how to hold babies to the breast and recognise the signs that they are properly attached and transferring a good flow of milk. There is now a strong evidence base on how babies transfer the milk and the optimum positions to hold and attach babies to achieve this. Unfortunately, many well-meaning families and professionals have thought that babies breastfeed in a similar way to sucking from bottles and it is just a matter of substituting one for the other. I will look at breastfeeding positions parents find comfortable, as well as the principles of attachment which you need to know in your practice with new parents. This chapter will explain the international initiatives to reinstate this knowledge and how the UK have responded to this.

Towards the end of the last century, it was becoming apparent globally that a crisis was arising in many societies as knowledge and practice of breastfeeding was being lost to families, despite it being the way babies had been fed since the beginning of mankind. An urgent need internationally to improve the skills of professionals caring for women was identified. The rise in the bottle-feeding culture and the actions of companies manufacturing, promoting and advertising formula milks meant that it was imperative to restore this knowledge.

In response to this crisis, and the publication of the Innocenti Declaration in 1991,[1] the Baby Friendly Hospital Initiative (BHFI)[2] was developed by the WHO and UNICEF in 1991, to implement practices that protect, promote and support breastfeeding. BFHI focusses on maternity services, and set out the 'Ten Steps to Successful Breastfeeding', the basic guidelines that staff needed to follow in order to offer parents the support and guidance they might need to initiate and maintain breastfeeding. It was introduced to the UK in 1995. The Ten Steps were reviewed in 2016 by WHO and UNICEF in the light of a systematic review of the evidence, which included 58 studies demonstrating the impact the Ten Steps had on the early initiation, exclusivity and duration of breastfeeding.[3] The steps were expanded to include critical management procedures as well as key clinical skills.

These critical management procedures comprise: ensuring compliance with the International Code of Marketing of Breastmilk Substitutes (discussed in Chapter 3); having an infant feeding policy that is routinely communicated to all staff; monitoring of data and ensuring staff have knowledge, competence and skills to support breastfeeding. Achieving these requires NHS management and university commitment.

DOI: 10.4324/9781003139775-5

I have also discussed the way Unicef UK Baby Friendly Initiative (BFI) in Chapter 3 has led the way globally by moving its focus towards a more holistic approach of supporting parents to build close and loving relationships with their babies. Here I will look at how hospital and community trusts and universities can follow a structured path to become Baby Friendly accredited by establishing policies and training staff to support parents with evidence-based information, to enable them to breastfeed their babies for as long as they planned and build close relationships with their babies.

How many NHS Trusts and universities are now UNICEF Baby Friendly accredited in the UK?

The Unicef UK Baby Friendly Initiative (BFI) had its original focus in 1991 on maternity services by following the Ten-Steps programme to support and encourage mothers to breastfeed and uphold the International Code of Marketing of Breastmilk Substitutes. Soon after this, the Seven Point Plan was introduced to embrace community as well as maternity services.

A major review of its standards was published in the UK in 2012, alongside the expanding evidence base, to encompass the wider benefits of breastfeeding in its role of increasing mothering hormones and building relationships between mothers and babies. These new Baby Friendly standards are specifically for UK settings and have led the world in changing the emphasis from primarily practical skills to relationship-building and include emotional support for parents who wish to bottle-feed formula to their babies. More recently, the standards have expanded to include skills for staff working in neonatal units, children's centres and universities.[4] Also, learning objectives and outcomes for other staff working with families and babies, such as medical students,[5] dietitians and pharmacists have been produced, with some accompanying training modules.

Many of you may be working in a community setting or be studying in a university which is UNICEF Baby Friendly accredited or working towards it. You are likely to have received the 'Relationship Building' training, which will have given you a basic evidence base and some vital skills to support parents with breastfeeding and building close, loving relationships with their babies.[6]

Some university courses training midwives have moved quickly to implement the UNICEF Baby Friendly training and to date 44% have become Baby Friendly accredited (January 2021), with 72% working towards it. Courses training health visitors have been slower to include the standards in their programmes, with only 17% fully accredited, but 28% working towards it. Hopefully, in the next few years more universities will achieve this standard so that new health visitors will be able to start their professional journey with these basic skills to support breastfeeding families.

More recently, BFI has implemented a higher qualification of breastfeeding. A Gold award has been introduced for units already accredited to achieve sustainability for excellent and sustained practices in maternity and community settings in support of infant feeding and parent–infant relationships. At the time of writing, 28 gold awards have been made.

The National Institute of Care Excellence (NICE)[7] recognised these skills in 2006 as reaching a minimum standard of breastfeeding support but, in order to be confident in supporting mothers with more complex issues, further breastfeeding training is required. In-service training should be available in your trust, sometimes run by your infant feeding coordinator, a breastfeeding counsellor or a lactation consultant.

The NHS long-term plan launched in January 2019 recognised the importance of breastfeeding standards in maternity units and stated:

All maternity services that do not deliver an accredited, evidence-based infant feeding programme, such as the Unicef Baby Friendly Initiative, will begin the accreditation process in 2019/20. Only 57% of babies in England are currently born in an accredited 'Baby Friendly' environment. Our breastfeeding rates compare unfavourably with other countries in Europe. There is substantial variation between parts of England, with 84% of children breastfed at 6–8 weeks in London compared to 32% in the North East.[8]

The Chief Midwife announced last year (2020) that there would be some funding available for maternity units not yet on the journey to become baby friendly to enable them to work towards becoming Baby Friendly accredited.

Questions expectant parents may ask you

If you are able to have face-to-face contacts with expectant parents, this is a perfect time to discuss breastfeeding and answer questions they may have. It is important to use the communication skills outlined in the last chapter to establish what they already know about feeding babies, by listening to them, before imparting any information. They may have heard from friends that it is difficult to help a baby to latch on the breast, or that sore nipples are normal and that bottle-feeding formula is just as good and more reliable. After listening to their questions, you will be able to offer them information which will help them gain confidence in breastfeeding as a feasible and healthy option.

Amazingly, if you listen attentively, they will usually give you openings to talk about why breastfeeding is important for babies' and mothers' health, some basic information about their baby's behaviour after birth and how to position and help babies follow their instincts when attaching to their breasts. Discussing new-born babies' behaviour can help parents' understanding of how frequently their baby will be wanting cuddles and reassurance, as well as feeding. Starting with skin-to skin contact after birth and 'rooming in' (keeping mothers and babies together after birth) enables the first and subsequent breastfeeds to happen through this close physical and emotional connection between mother and baby. Expectant parents may also ask how they can prepare themselves before their babies' birth (Figure 5.1, 5.2).

Preparation before birth

Can I hand express and store colostrum when pregnant?

Hand expressing is a skill and the technique can be demonstrated easily with a knitted breast antenatally. Hand expressing antenatally can help women get used to handling their breasts. Both parents can gain confidence in breastfeeding by seeing drops of colostrum coming out of the woman's nipples!

Usually women wait until 36 week's gestation before they begin expressing, as it was previously thought there was a theoretical risk of stimulating premature labour through the release of oxytocin, but this fear is not backed up by research.[9] Women who have a history of premature labour may still be advised to wait as late as possible before attempting to do it. Many midwives suggest that women 'harvest colostrum' to build a

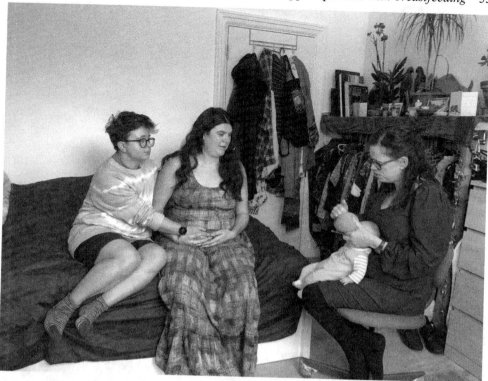

Figure 5.1 Antenatal contact at home

supply in their freezers, especially if they have gestational or Type 1 or 2 diabetes. The reason for this is that their babies are more vulnerable to having unstable blood sugars after birth and additional colostrum can be given to stabilise these instead of formula milk. The added advantage of giving colostrum is that it will protect the baby's microbiome, gut bacteria and immunity. Other women may choose to harvest colostrum in case their babies have problems latching on their breasts after birth. Midwives will usually give women a supply of the purple oral syringes (1 or 2ml) with bungs, in which they can collect and store the frozen colostrum. This ensures there is no wastage, because the defrosted colostrum can be given directly to the baby by removing the bung and putting it between the baby's lips into the corner of her mouth.

How do I express and store colostrum?

1   The woman can begin by gently massaging her breasts with her hands, after a warm shower or after applying warm compresses. She could then gently touch or roll her nipples. This stimulates the nerve endings, which will send messages to the pituitary gland in her brain to release oxytocin, which will trigger some colostrum to flow down the ducts in her breasts towards her nipples (see Figure 5.3).
2   She can make a C-shape, cupping her breast with her hand, her fingers underneath and thumb on top. If she walks her thumb from the base of the nipple, she will feel the breast tissue underneath change from the nipple to areola. She will discover a

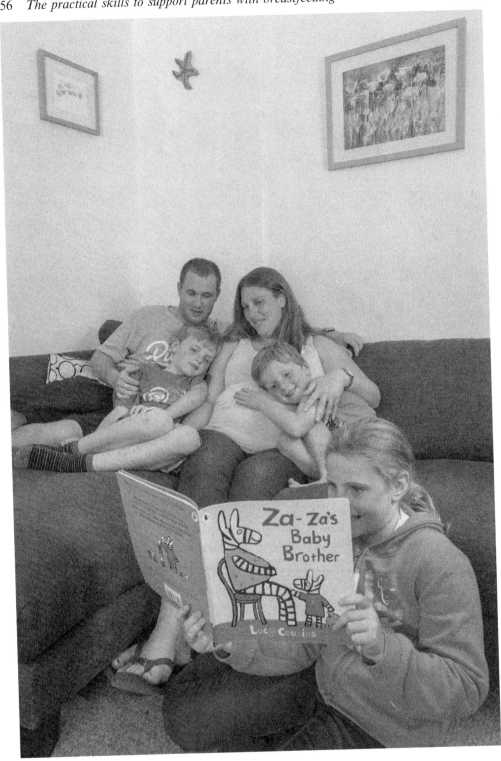

Figure 5.2 Expectant family
Source: Images supplied by Real Baby Milk, a project of Pollen CIC.

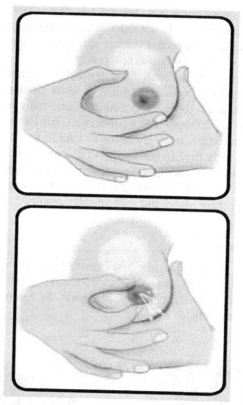

Figure 5.3 Hand expressing
Source: Courtesy of Start4Life.

      lumpier area behind, usually on the margin of the areola and breast tissue, which is the position to express.

3   She can then move her thumb down on to the lumpy area in a slightly backwards direction on to the breast tissue underneath and at the same time move her fingers upwards from below and apply gentle pressure. It is important to hold this for 4–5 seconds to allow the sticky colostrum drops to come out of the nipple.

4   It is common the first time she tries for nothing to come out of the nipple! This probably indicates that she needs to try to stimulate the oxytocin release again by warm compresses and gentle massaging.

5   Hand expressing is a skill and may be hard to start with, but if she perseveres it will become easier. There are videos on YouTube on harvesting colostrum which can be very helpful.

Possible questions after birth

Why is skin-to-skin so important after the birth?

Babies have strong instinctive behaviour immediately after birth and, if mothers can follow their baby's lead, they can start their breastfeeding journey.

Most expectant parents have heard that they will be offered skin-to-skin with their babies immediately after birth, but perhaps do not know why it is so important (Figure 5.4). In the last ten years in the UK there has been a change in maternity care, with all hospitals now enabling parents to get to know their babies in this way.

It is through this close contact with their mother that close, loving relationships develop between mothers and babies, resulting in some paediatricians and psychologists using the term 'the dyad' to describe a mother and baby being in tune with each other and acting as one unit. Through this connection, babies and mothers produce the 'love' hormone oxytocin, which not only helps to stimulate the mother's 'let down' in her breasts, making her milk flow to her baby, but also gives them both a warm feeling of closeness. Thus, breastfeeding is not just about health. Fathers and partners also make oxytocin when cuddling their babies close, especially when they have skin-to-skin contact, which will help them also build a close relationship.

What is the 'breast crawl'?

Immediately after birth, babies take their first breaths but may not cry much if the birth was gentle. The midwife will dry the baby, but may leave some amniotic fluid on their hands, which may help guide the baby to the breast, as a mother's colostrum has a similar smell to her breastmilk.

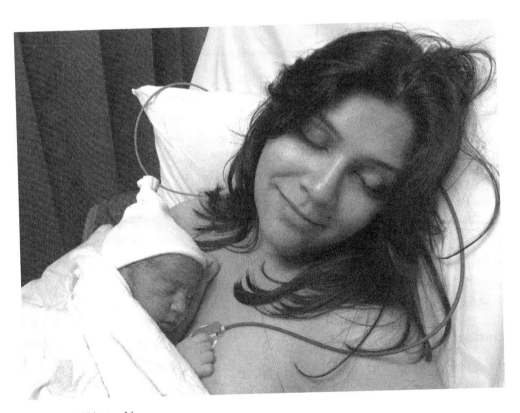

Figure 5.4 Skin-to-skin

Babies will be placed directly on their mother's abdomen, after a vaginal delivery, or on to her chest after a caesarean section. There they begin their 'breast crawl' towards her breasts. In this *golden hour* after birth, babies go through distinct phases while mothers' and babies' bodies and brains begin to respond to each other and develop deep connections.

Babies are stronger than we think. It may be tempting to help them, but letting them find the breasts themselves, so following what nature intended them to do, appears to imprint breastfeeding behaviour which they will follow at subsequent feeds. They have instinctive behaviour which helps them find the breasts for themselves, and parents begin to realise that babies know what to do!

The first phase is a time of relaxation while the infant rests, listens to the familiar sounds from his mother's body and recovers from the birth. This may last for some time, while his parents gaze and marvel at their new baby. Next there is an awakening phase when he begins to show signs of activity and starts to move his head up and down and from side to side and make small movements with his limbs. This is followed by an active phase as he makes larger movements, pushes with his arms and legs and begins 'rooting' movements with his head bobbing up and down and side to side. The 'crawling' motions then begin as baby starts to draw up his legs with the knees bent and then push with his feet, so propelling himself up his mother's body towards her breasts.

The baby may then rest again and may start sucking on his hands. Once he is near her breasts, he might then brush against her nipples with his cheeks and start to lick her nipple, sometimes moving from one breast to the other. Amazingly he knows there are two breasts! He may rest again before rooting, opening his mouth wide like a big yawn, he scoops the nipple and areola up with his tongue, drawing it to the back of his mouth, takes a large mouthful of breast and starts sucking.

The mother's body will also produce a surge of hormones as her baby starts feeding and she begins to smell, stroke and look at her new baby as she relaxes after the birth.

Is skin-to-skin only important if parents want to breastfeed?

Skin-to-skin can help babies at any time, whether they are breast or bottle fed, especially in the first few months when they are stressed or struggling to latch on their mothers' breasts, or just want a close cuddle. Fathers or partners can have skin-to-skin with their new babies immediately after birth if mothers require medical intervention, until they are able to do it. If they wish to breastfeed, then it is very helpful that mothers have skin-to-skin as soon as possible, but all parents can enjoy this special time, whether they intend to breastfeed or not. (Figure 5.5).

As well as enabling the first breastfeed, an amazing connection develops between parents' and babies' bodies and brains. Research done on preterm babies when kept skin-to-skin or in 'kangaroo mother care' (KMC), has found that, incredibly, if the baby is cold, the mother's body temperature rises and, if the baby is too warm, her body cools him/her down; this is called 'thermo-synchrony'.[10] Babies are so relaxed when skin-to-skin with one of their parents that their breathing is regulated, heart rate slows, blood pressure lowers and, because they are not burning up their body reserve fuels, their blood sugars remain stable; they maintain homeostasis better. KMC with preterm babies improves their sleep, neurodevelopment and growth, and their emotional connection (attachment) with parents happens more easily.

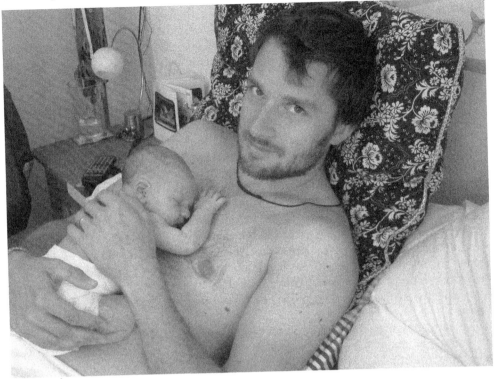

Figure 5.5 A father enjoying skin-to-skin contact

It is relatively recently that babies have been separated from their mothers after birth in Western societies, but in many countries in the world babies and mothers still remain together after birth and cots are not used. This separation we often have in the UK after birth can have a detrimental effect on the way a mother responds to her baby's feeding cues because she may not notice the early signs of her baby's restlessness or sucking of hands. These may indicate that her baby is hungry, especially when her baby is lying in a cot some distance from her. Responding to babies' early feeding cues will enable the baby to latch on the breast more easily. Brain scans have shown that connections are built in a baby's emotional centres while relaxing in this close contact, which I will be discussing in the chapter on mental health. After this first breastfeed, babies often fall into a long, deep sleep, content after their first colostrum feed, and, if they are assessed to be healthy, it seems important not to disturb them from this restorative sleep.

How can I hold my baby for breastfeeding?

Parents are likely to want information from you before the birth and at the first postnatal visit on how to hold their baby to enable effective attachment. In many countries where breastfeeding is the normal way babies are fed, people may find this question strange, because they have grown up seeing it around them. In Western countries, babies being breastfed are not commonly seen in public places. Women may try to imitate bottle-feeding techniques by holding their babies in the crook of their arms and 'posting' their breasts into the centre of their babies' mouth. This does not work as the nipples are usually too central in the babies' mouths and they cannot draw them back towards their soft palates. The nipples may also rub on their hard palates and become sore and damaged.

You can demonstrate how to hold their babies with a doll and a knitted breast, which you could keep in your bag, This learned or imitated behaviour from bottle-feeding will not only cause the mother pain but the baby is unlikely to get much milk, because the nipple is in the centre of the baby's mouth, not far in (shallow latch) rather than high in the mouth and deeply in (deep latch). The way the mother holds her baby will make a difference to the way the baby can access the breast to gain a good flow of milk.

As well as offering parents some suggestions on how they could hold their babies for breastfeeding, you could also give them some visual materials or leaflets to illustrate this, or links to online videos, to reinforce the learning. If mothers can achieve effective attachment at the breast right from birth, they can avoid most of the common problems. Any baby who is still hungry after feeds or gaining less weight than expected is likely to benefit from better positioning so that he can achieve an effective latch and good milk flow.

What are the principles of positioning babies for breastfeeding?

For those of you who have already done the UNICEF BFI training this will be a revision, but it is always useful to re-visit it. I will outline different breastfeeding positions and what happens to the baby's mouth when they attach effectively to obtain good milk transfer. This is the most important information parents will need because it does not come to mothers instinctively.

These helpful tips apply to all breastfeeding positions and they can help to guide parents on how to hold babies in the optimum way. The acronym CHIN helps with remembering some basic points:

C – Close
H – head free
I – in line
N – nose to nipple

Close means that the baby's body is held very close to and touching his mother's body. Many mothers do not realise how close they need to hold their babies for breastfeeding.

Head free – babies' heads need to be free to tilt backwards, so they can open their mouth wide and come to the breast with their chin leading. Parents often want to hold the back of the baby's heads, because they are floppy after birth and do not have good head control. By putting a hand behind their baby's shoulders and under their ears, a mother can support her baby's head well. If someone held the back of your head when you are trying to drink you would not be able to take a mouthful or swallow the fluid!

In-line means that babies' bodies are held in a straight line without twisting and their heads, shoulders, hips and legs are in a line.

Nose to nipple – babies are brought to the breast with their nose level with their mother's nipple. Mothers may be tempted to move their breasts towards their babies, but this will make their nipples too central in their babies' mouths, rather than towards their top lips and the roofs of their mouths.

When might parents ask about breastfeeding positions?

You could discuss holding the baby for breastfeeding with them in general at the antenatal contact, but discuss different positions in more detail at your new baby contact as you will be doing a feeding assessment, and can listen to their breastfeeding journey. Using the communication skills described in the last chapter, you can ask about their experiences of the birth of the baby. A vaginal delivery seems to set up the breastfeeding hormones in the mother, whereas a caesarean section might take a bit longer. If she has had an epidural, or other drugs, there is some evidence to suggest they could delay the release of prolactin and oxytocin.[11]

What are the cradle and cross-cradle positions?

These are the most commonly used positions and ones that some parents may have already seen mothers using in public places, or portrayed in classical art. Some mothers

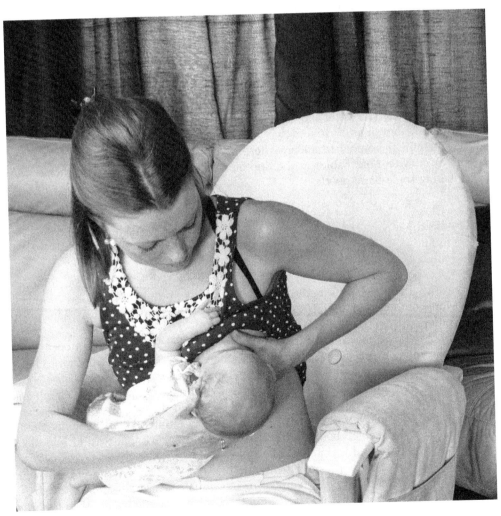

Figure 5.6 Cross-cradle position
Source: Images supplied by Real Baby Milk, a project of Pollen CIC.

will often start their breastfeeding journey by using the cross-cradle position, to ensure the baby's head is tilted back and mouth wide open so they can take a large mouthful of the lower areola with their tongue and lower jaw (see Figure 5.6 and 5.8) Their chin

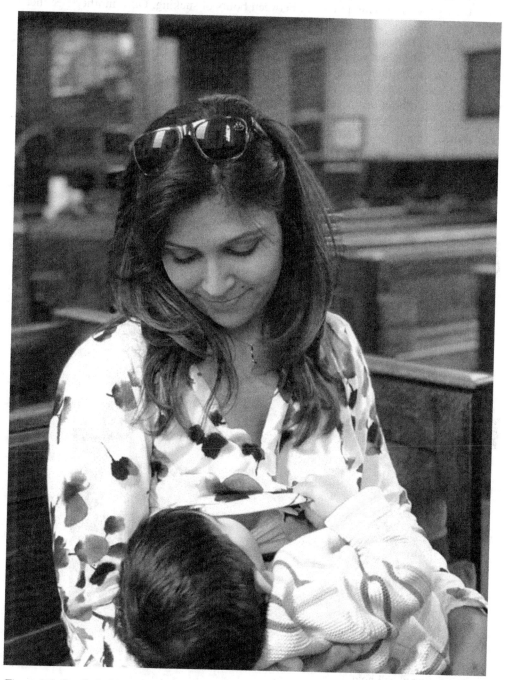

Figure 5.7 Cradle hold

should be indenting the breasts while they draw their nipple along the roof of their mouth almost to the junction with the soft palate and begin to take small sucks.

When babies are feeding well and the milk is flowing, following the let down (triggered by the release of oxytocin), babies begin to do long, drawing sucks with swallows, using their jaws and having pauses in between bouts of sucking. Once mothers see their baby is well attached and can hear their baby swallowing, they often move their other arm across into the cradle position to support the weight of the baby, and may then put a cushion or pillow for support under their arm. I usually suggest that it is better to position and attach their baby first, before bringing a cushion, in to support their arm. Some mothers who use breastfeeding cushions or pillows from the beginning may find their baby is too high up to latch effectively, especially as they get older. Many babies attach to the breast better if their body is held lower, often at an angle of 45 degrees to their mother's body (see Figures 5.7 and 5.8).

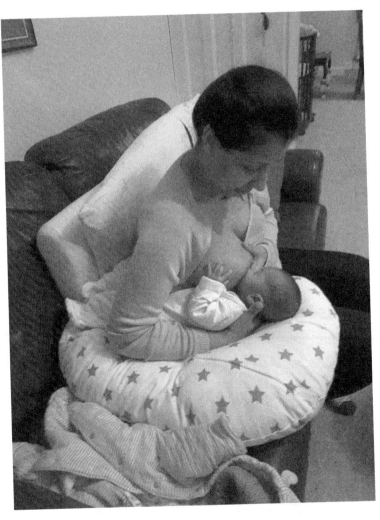

Figure 5.8 Rubgy ball hold

What is the 'rugby ball' hold?

It is called this because it resembles the way rugby players hold the ball! (see Figure 5.8) This position can be very helpful when a baby is small or premature, the mother's breasts are large, her nipples are flat or inverted or she has had a caesarean and does not want pressure on her lower abdomen by her scar. The baby's body can be held at her side, below her breast, with his/her legs protruding behind her, making sure that the principles of CHIN are followed. Some mothers prefer to have a pillow behind their backs, so there is room for baby's legs and a small cushion under their baby's body. She holds her baby close to her body, making sure the head is free to tilt back by supporting behind the baby's shoulders with the hand on the same side. The baby's body needs to be in a straight line and not twisted and held with his/her nose level with the mother's nipple (without moving her breast).

What is the side-lying position?

This position is not usually the first one that women use at the beginning of breast-feeding, as it is a little harder to master. If a mother has stitches in her perineum, this can be less painful as she will not be sitting on them. The mother lies on her side with her baby lying on his/her side facing her, body close, in a straight line (see Figure 5.9). She brings the baby towards her breast with his/her neck extended backwards and, the baby's nose level with her nipple, leading with his chin. A difficulty that mothers sometimes find with this position is that they are holding their baby too high in relation to their body so may find it easier if they move their baby lower, enabling the baby to extend their head further back, and look up at them.

How can we use the laid-back position? ('Biological Nurturing')

The mother can lie on a sofa or bed in a semi-reclining position with her baby lying on top of her, either in skin-to-skin contact or with clothes on (see Figure 5.10). This position has probably been used by mothers around the world for thousands of years, as they rest and recover from their births, but it was described in Europe more recently by Suzanne Colson as 'Biological Nurturing'.[12] She suggested that mothers lay back and their babies lie on top of their bodies with their body contours fitting into their mothers' bodies, rather than adopting a regimented way of latching their babies on their breasts. Babies then tend to behave in an instinctive way similar to the way they do after birth during skin-to-skin contact. They smell their mother's milk and start to search for the breast by moving their heads from side to side and opening their mouths wider and wider, until they find the nipple and areola and latch on themselves. This position can be helpful for babies who are struggling in the early days to attach effectively to the breast. She says in referring to her book that:

> The challenge for health professionals lies with promoting an oxytocin-friendly environment, understanding breastfeeding releasing mechanisms, and learning when not to intervene. This book restores confidence in nature's biological design and in mothers' innate capacity to breastfeed.[13]

A variation of biological nurturing, sometimes called the koala position, is when mothers are sitting up with babies held in an upright position, facing

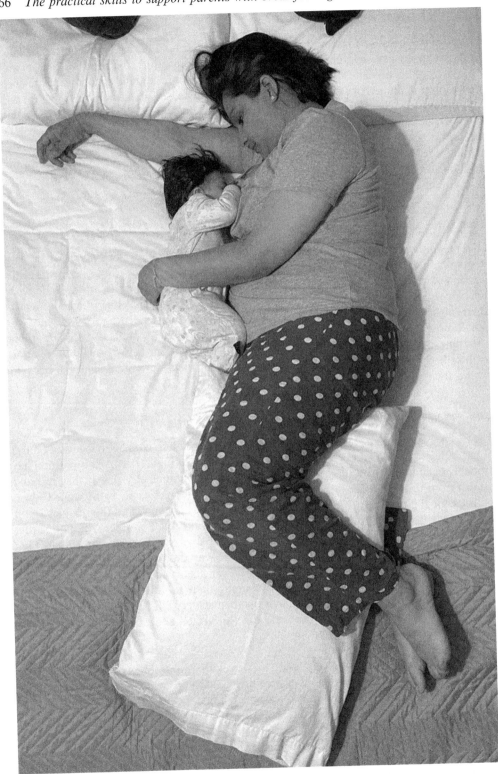

Figure 5.9 Side-lying position

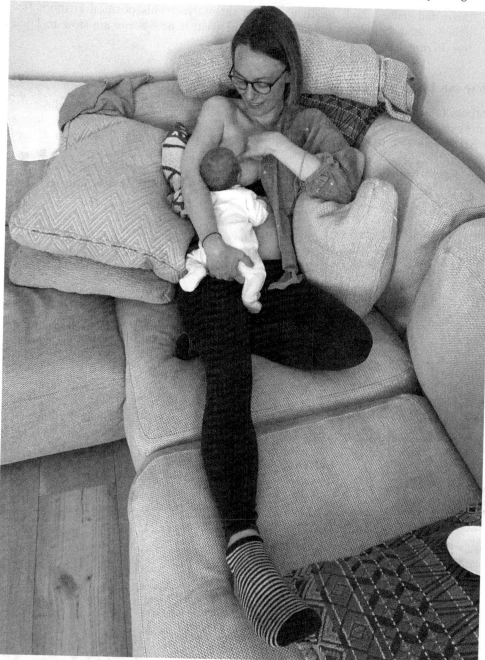

Figure 5.10 Biological nurturing/laid-back position
Source: Cordelia Uys.

them and babies latch on their breasts themselves. This position is more frequently used with older babies, but can be tried if new-borns are slow to latch (see Figure 5.11).

How can I help my baby latch on to my breast?

Parents in the UK are often not prepared for this deep attachment in which the baby's mouth cavity is completely full of breast tissue, because they probably have a visual image of bottle feeding with the baby just taking the teat into the middle of his mouth.

Every mother and baby dyad is different, but the way a baby is held and latches on to the breast largely determines the volume of breastmilk that is transferred to

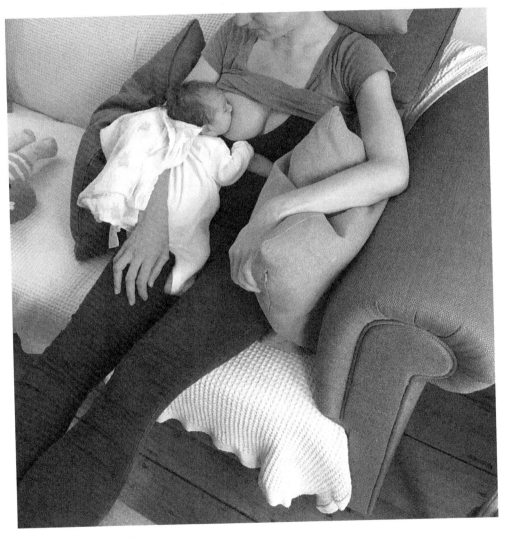

Figure 5.11 Koala hold
Source: Cordelia Uys.

him. When he is brought to the breast with his nose level with his mother's nipple, he will smell the colostrum/milk, start to root (turn his head from side to side) and open his mouth. When his mouth is very wide, like a yawn, the mother can bring him to her breast quickly with his chin touching the breast first, the lower lip probably level with the edge of the lower areola (depending on the size of the areola), and the nipple aimed towards his top lip. Then the baby draws the nipple to the roof of his mouth with his tongue, which stimulates the sucking reflex, and he draws it nearly all the way back to the junction of his hard and soft palate. Once the baby has opened his mouth wide, his mother needs to move his body rapidly towards hers, with his chin touching first. As her baby draws her nipple to the back of his mouth, he takes a large mouthful which fills his mouth cavity with breast tissue.[14]

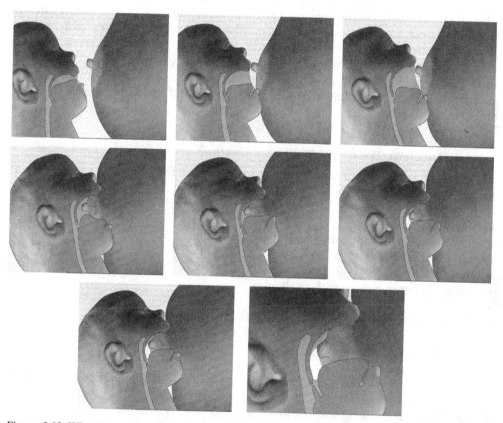

Figure 5.12 What happens in a baby's mouth as they attach. Images from the Baby Buddy app, courtesy of Best Beginnings. Baby Buddy 2.0 is a parenting app with daily information updates for mums, dads and co-parents. It supports families every step of the way through pregnancy and until the child's first birthday with evidence-based articles and videos. It is free and advert-free and can be accessed from Google and Apple App Stores: https://www.babybuddyapp.co.uk/.[15]

How do we tell if babies are well latched on the breasts?

Once the baby is attached to his mother's breast in this optimum way, the whole of his mouth is full of breast tissue, with the nipple resting high in his mouth near the junction of hard and soft palate and he will begin to feed, following a certain pattern.

Initially, he will take a few small, shallow sucks to stimulate the release of oxytocin (the 'love' hormone) which triggers his mother's let-down reflex and makes the milk flow through the ducts in her breast towards her nipples. Then the baby begins to have bouts of slow, drawing sucks, using his jaws making a ripple movement with his tongue, moving the colostrum/milk towards the back of his mouth so he can swallow it. He will have short pauses between bouts of sucking.

Once he has finished feeding on that breast, he will usually release the suction and move his head away. Sometimes babies may fall asleep and release the breast when they have finished that breast. They will often take the second breast after a few minutes but some are satisfied with one breast, particularly in the early weeks. It is worth offering the other breast at each feed unless the baby is clearly already full. It is important to reassure mothers that their breasts are never empty and there is always more for a second, third or more helpings! When a baby re-latches, another let down will happen as the baby sucks and more breastmilk will be available.

What does my baby look like when attached effectively on my breast?

These points will be useful for parents to look for and for you when you observe a mother breastfeeding (see Figure 5.13).

- mouth open wide
- more areola visible at baby's nose than baby's chin
- chin indenting breast, gap for nose
- fully puffed cheeks
- deep, rhythmic sucking with swallows
- no pain!
- (there may be a little discomfort in the first 15 seconds of the feed)

To ensure good attachment:

- his mother moves him quickly to her breast with a wide mouth (like a yawn with his tongue down)
- his chin touches the breast first and her nipple is level with his top lip
- he scoops the lower areola and nipple up with his tongue and draws the nipple back nearly to the junction of his soft palate
- his mouth cavity is full of breast tissue
- his latch is asymmetrical because there is more areola above his top lip than below his bottom lip
- he takes a few quick sucks which trigger the let down
- he does long jaw movements with audible swallows followed by pauses.

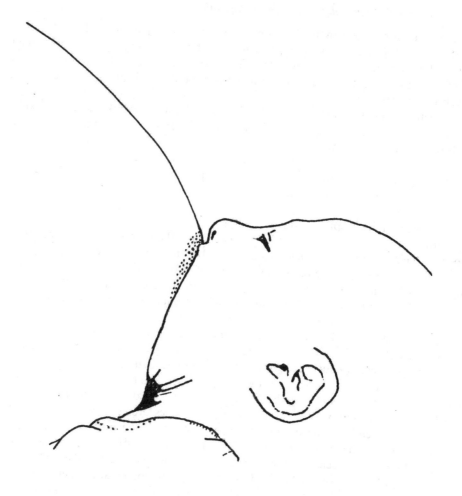

Figure 5.13 Well attached
Source: Line drawing by Jenny Richardson

Will I make enough milk for my baby?

We are mammals and as such nature intended us to breastfeed our babies! Many pregnant women may worry whether their bodies will make enough milk for their babies and surveys have indicated that this is a common concern.[16] Families may lack confidence in the reliability of her breastmilk supply so are unable to reassure her. You can give explanations about how to stimulate and maintain the breastmilk supply. Mothers can assess whether their babies are latching effectively on to their breasts and their babies are transferring milk by listening to swallows. If babies are breastfeeding frequently and effectively, almost all women will make plenty of milk for them. Some paediatricians use the term '4th trimester of pregnancy' as human babies are very immature at birth and need the special nutrients and protection from disease that colostrum and breastmilk confer.

How can we tell if our baby is getting enough milk?

The volume of milk a baby is receiving worries most new parents and families because they cannot measure what is going in with breastfeeding, unlike bottle feeding! Understanding the way babies achieve effective transfer of milk, before their babies are born, will give parents the confidence to position and attach them and recognise how much they are taking.

At your antenatal contact, you could give them a leaflet or links to reliable websites, or apps, or demonstrate with a doll and a knitted breast. Communicating this bodily skill sensitively is not always easy, and for some parents there may be cultural reasons why it may not be appropriate to discuss this with fathers-to-be. If you give them sources of information, they can review them privately afterwards. Their family and friends may not be able to reassure them because they have no experience of breastfeeding.

New-born babies display frequent feeding cues, indicating they want to breastfeed, by turning their heads from side to side, putting their hand in their mouths, and opening their mouths wide. Their parents may be surprised by how often they want to feed, which is usually more often than formula-fed babies because they take longer to digest formula milk. They do this to fill their small stomachs and, usefully, at the same time this builds up their mother's milk supply by increasing the prolactin, so establishing the 'supply and demand'.

After the baby has taken a feed on the first breast, she will usually come off, or fall asleep and look relaxed and satisfied. She may then wake up again in a few minutes, start displaying feeding cues such as rooting, which indicate that she would like some more milk, so her mother can move her to the second breast. She may take a shorter feed here and fall asleep or may want to go back on a breast for a third or fourth time afterwards.

When parents are responding to their baby's feeding cues, even if they seem to come to the breast very frequently at the beginning, this will stimulate the mothers' milk supply by making high prolactin and oxytocin levels, which means they will continue to produce plenty of milk in the coming weeks, months and years. Frequent breastfeeds in the early weeks are very important and the parents will need to reassure any doubting family members!

Sometimes mothers have strong let downs causing rapid milk flow as oxytocin is released at the beginning of the feed. The baby may have problems keeping up with the speed of the milk and come off the breast coughing! This may happen if the mother's breasts are very full in the early weeks of the baby's life. As the milk is removed, the pressure reduces, the flow slows down and the baby can breastfeed happily again.

The way the baby feeds on the breast will tell parents if he is well attached and achieving good milk transfer. They can hear the milk going down! When he is well attached, he starts taking some short, quick sucks to stimulate his mother's oxytocin release. This hormone acts in the breast lactiferous tissue by squeezing the muscular epithelial cells around the milk-producing acini cells, which moves the milk down the ducts towards the nipple. His sucking then changes to a long, drawing action where he uses his jaws while ripples in his tongue move the milk towards the back of his mouth (see Figure 5.14).

In the first 2–3 days, parents will hear clicks in his throat as he swallows small amounts of colostrum. However, towards the end of the first week, the volume of mature milk increases, so louder gulps will be heard as he swallows more. Following this active phase, the number of bouts of sucking become less and pauses will become longer so parents may think that their babies are falling asleep because often their eyes

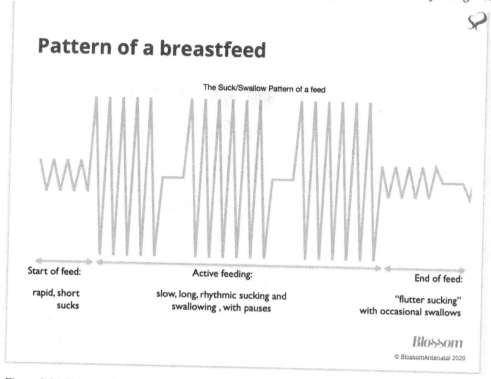

Figure 5.14 Pattern of a breastfeed.
Source: Drawing courtesy of Blossom Antenatal

are closed. There is no need to stroke their faces or toes to try to keep them awake (unless they are sleepy, premature or jaundiced) because their mothers are likely to have another let down and the milk will flow again. Then the baby will start drawing the milk again by using their jaw and tongue and swallowing will be heard again. We need to trust babies to follow their instincts!

What can new-born babies' nappies tell us?

Apart from watching how the baby feeds on the breast, parents can take note of what comes out in their baby's nappies and how this changes during the first week. This will reassure them and give them confidence that their baby is taking adequate volumes of milk. A full breastfeed should be observed and possible adjustments suggested if needed to the baby's positioning and attachment. By the time their baby is 5 days old, if he is passing at least two yellow stools which are larger than a £2 coin, (not just spotting) and five wet nappies, and he is contented after feeds, it would indicate that he is receiving plenty of milk (see Figure 5.15). The midwife will usually weigh him at 5 days when she also does the blood spot test. Most babies lose weight in the first 2–3 days after birth, following a fluid balance adjustment from placental life. This weight loss will be addressed later in Chapter 8, but just to say here that most babies lose less than 8% of their birthweight. If they lose any more than the threshold of 10%, the positioning and attachment should be checked, to optimise the milk transfer.

Newborn Nappy Output

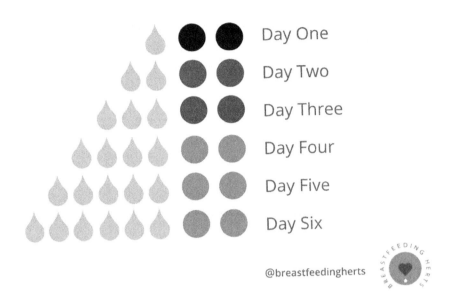

Figure 5.15 What is in a nappy
Source: Image supplied by Heidi Hembry IBCLC

How does a mother's breastmilk change in the first weeks after birth?

In the first few days after birth the colostrum is present in small volumes, starting with about 5–10 mls a feed on the first day. This fills the baby's stomach, which is about the size of a cherry, so satisfying her hunger.

Colostrum is often referred to as 'liquid gold' because of its high value to the baby, but it is not always yellow! It can be various colours including greenish, grey or blood-stained (known as 'rusty pipe'!). It is very high in protein due to the antibodies present, which provide babies with some protection against all the diseases the mother has had or been immunised against in her life, as well as giving babies all the nutrition they need. It also continues to build the baby's gut microbiome, a process which began at birth, and coats the gaps on the inside of the intestines like a 'white paint', sealing them to prevent bacteria and viruses from entering the baby's body. This helps in setting up the child with good health prospects for the rest of his life.

Do babies want to breastfeed only when they are hungry?

Babies breastfeed when they are hungry or thirsty, but also when they want a cuddle, to be comforted or reassured, or lulled into sleep. Babies love breastfeeding and appear to be in a wonderful, dreamy state afterwards! Some refer to this as looking 'milk drunk'! Many mothers also enjoy this special close time with their babies, which is not governed by the clock, but the flow of milk passing between them, a natural time, not unlike the flowing of rivers. Through this responsive feeding, mothers and babies build up close relationships as their bodies and brains work together, giving them both, through their oxytocin release, a profound sense of well-being and closeness. I will discuss in the next chapter how this leads to empathic attachment between mother and baby, with good mental health outcomes for both of them.

I have argued in Chapter 10 that this mechanistic word 'breastfeeding' may limit understanding of the process, because it implies that the only function is the transfer of milk, whereas it is so much more. It does not encompass the whole experience for mothers and babies, when they are responding to each other physically and emotionally, building a closeness that will last a lifetime. Other languages have broader words for breastfeeding, such as 'nursing' in the USA and 'stillen' in German, which means 'restful', suggesting more of a calming, parenting relationship. You cannot overfeed or 'spoil' a baby by breastfeeding responsively! Despite what others may be saying!

Will I need to buy a breast pump?

When a baby is breastfeeding effectively there is no need to buy a pump, unless it is for certain specific situations, such as when parents want to give expressed milk from a bottle. The other important reasons for using a pump will be if the mother is separated from her baby who needs to be nursed in a special care baby unit, or if her baby is not latching onto her breasts. In these cases, using a hospital grade breast pump, at least eight times in 24 hours (including in the middle of the night, when she is making most milk) will provide her baby with her very valuable colostrum and breastmilk and at the same time stimulate her milk supply. In the case of a preterm baby, her milk will provide specific ingredients to suit his/her stage of gestation. Mother's breasts always know the age of her baby! As I discussed in Chapter 2, breastmilk will help to protect her baby from the very dangerous bowel condition necrotising enterocolitis (NEC). Many pump manufacturers hire hospital grade, double breast pumps, which are the most effective ones, and this works out much cheaper. Double pumping means that mothers can express both breasts simultaneously and this may increase the volume collected, rather than pumping from each breast in turn.

When can my partner give expressed milk from a bottle?

Many partners understandably want to share the feeding experience and give their babies expressed milk from bottles. Perhaps you could suggest that this is delayed until the baby is about 4–6 weeks old, so the mother's milk supply has adjusted to meet her baby's needs and breastfeeding technique has been established. At this age, babies are able to adjust to feeding from bottles as well as breasts, but if parents leave it much later, many babies will refuse to take a bottle. Using a 'paced' bottle-feeding technique may help to slow the milk flow down as parents respond to their baby's behaviour. Here babies take the teats into their mouths by rooting and drawing them in, with the bottle held horizontally. The bottle can then be tipped more vertically to allow the teat to fill with milk and then returned to a horizontal position. In this way babies respond to the milk flow but do not get overwhelmed with too much. They have pauses in between bouts of sucking, in a similar way to when they breastfeed. Partners often have more success giving their babies expressed milk from a bottle than mothers, because babies cannot smell milk on them!

What can I do if I cannot express my milk?

Some women find expressing harder than others but have plenty of milk for their babies. It is an artificial way of getting milk out of breasts, working by applying negative pressure around the nipple and areola. Many mothers' bodies do not respond to pumping, which needs the release of oxytocin (the 'love' hormone) to let down their milk. Most women do not fall in love with a bit of plastic! It may help for mothers to stimulate their breasts before using the pump, by applying warm compresses, or having a shower, gently massaging the breast and stroking the areola and nipples. Hand expressing can stimulate more oxytocin because of the sensation of touch on the breasts and may be worth doing for a few minutes before applying the breast pump. Obviously, the baby feeding is the best way to make the milk flow, so the best time to express is often straight after a breastfeed, or during a feed. Some pumps can be used while the baby is feeding on the other breast, by collecting milk at the same time. If mothers are expressing when their babies are in a neonatal unit, it can help to do so next to their incubators or have a photo of the baby beside them when doing so at home and express eight to ten times in 24 hours.

How do I know if my growing baby is getting enough milk?

Parents learn to understand their babies' feeding cues and know when they are indicating they want to breastfeed and can breastfeed responsively. After the first week of life, babies' breastfeeding techniques tend to become more efficient, displaying the suck–swallow pattern described above and swallows will be heard. Some babies may still be sleepy after the birth and not waking regularly for feeds, so parents will need to wake them up by changing their nappies before feeds and if this does not work, to hand express colostrum and feed with a syringe. Other babies may be alert and showing early feeding cues, which is the ideal time for mothers to breastfeed. They will indicate that they have finished the first breast when they come off decisively, looking relaxed, happy and full (milk drunk!) or some may fall asleep and gradually fall off the breast looking contented. After a period of time or after a nappy change, most babies begin to show feeding cues by 'rooting' and searching for the breast, opening their mouths. This is the time for mothers to offer their second breast and usually babies feed for shorter periods of time on them. This mother shared with me her story about unhelpful advice she received about only offering one breast a feed:

> I was told by a health visitor at six weeks that I should only feed on one side for each feed so that the breast would be fully drained. The reason for doing this was to ensure the hind milk would be reached and the baby would be full. This led to severe engorgement and discomfort and I contacted a lactation consultant for advice who told me that this was what was causing the engorgement and I should switch sides as required at each feed. Once I stopped doing this, things sorted themselves, out but I was annoyed to have such flawed advice.

There is usually no need to wind breastfed babies, or spend time patting their backs, because they do not usually swallow air when not coordinating their suck–swallow pattern well, but sometimes they may bring up burps, or small mouthfuls of milk (possets) when moved. Some babies will become efficient at breastfeeding and finish quickly, whereas others may take their time, but you cannot tell how much milk they have taken by the length of the feed.

As I said earlier, timing feeds is not important and does not indicate how much fore- or hindmilk the baby has taken. As soon as the let down works, the fatty content starts rising and babies decide when to finish the feed. The only way to tell how much the baby is taking is to look at the stools and urine output how contented she is and her weight gain. If she is taking a long time over feeds, is very fussy or is slow to regain her birthweight, it is likely that her milk transfer is not optimum and would benefit from a full feeding assessment, which includes a review of her positioning and attachment on the breast. Expected weight gain will be covered in Chapter 8 on weighing babies.

Why is optimum positioning and attachment so important?

Once a mother is confident about the way she holds her baby and he is latching effectively, feeds become more efficient, and babies more content. A frequent cause of babies not obtaining a good flow of milk is that they are not positioned or attached in an optimum way, which may be because mothers are bringing their babies to their breasts with their nipples too central in their mouths. An asymmetrical latch is very important to enable a baby to take a large mouthful of areola with her chin near the margin of the areola and breast, and her top lip resting over the top of the mother's nipple. It also prevents mothers from developing sore nipples, as they are not rubbing on the hard palate on the roofs of their babies' mouths, but are scooped up by their tongues and drawn along the top of their mouths close to the junction of the hard and soft palate, a place where they cannot be damaged. Breastfeeding will then become comfortable and enjoyable for both mother and baby.

Useful links:

https://globalhealthmedia.org/portfolio-items/breastfeeding-in-the-first-hours-after-birth/
https://globalhealthmedia.org/portfolio-items/continuous-skin-to-skin-care/
https://globalhealthmedia.org/portfolio-items/breastfeeding-attachment/
https://www.breastfeedingnetwork.org.uk/drugs-factsheets/
https://play.google.com/store/apps/details?id=uk.org.bestbeginnings.babybuddy&hl=en_GB&gl=US

Notes

1 UNICEF (1991) *Innocenti Declaration on the Protection, Promotion and Support of Breastfeeding*. Available at: www.unicef.org/nutrition/index_24807.html
2 WHO (1991) *Ten Steps to Successful Breastfeeding*. Available at: www.who.int/activities/promoting-baby-friendly-hospitals/ten-steps-to-successful-breastfeeding
3 Ibid.
4 UNICEF (2018) *History of Baby Friendly in the UK*. Available at: https://www.unicef.org.uk/babyfriendly/about/history/
5 UNICEF UK (2019) *Baby Friendly Initiative Learning Outcomes – Medical Students*. Available at: www.unicef.org.uk/babyfriendly/wp-content/uploads/sites/2/2019/07/Medical-student-learning-outcomes-guidance.pdf
6 UNICEF (2012) *Relationship Building Resources: Baby Friendly Initiative*. Available at: www.unicef.org.uk/babyfriendly/baby-friendly-resources/relationship-building-resources/
7 NICE (2021) *Overview:Postnatal Care – Guidance*. NICE. Available at: www.nice.org.uk/guidance/ng194

8　UNICEF (2019) *NHS Long Term Plan Recommends Baby Friendly*. Available at: www. unicef.org.uk/babyfriendly/nhs-long-term-plan-recommends-baby-friendly/

9　Forster, D. A. *et al.* (2017) 'Advising women with diabetes in pregnancy to express breastmilk in late pregnancy (Diabetes and Antenatal Milk Expressing [DAME]): A multicentre, unblinded, randomised controlled trial', *The Lancet*, 389(10085), pp. 2204–2213.

10　Campbell-Yeo, M. L. *et al.* (2015) 'Understanding kangaroo care and its benefits to preterm infants', *Pediatric Health, Medicine and Therapeutics*, 6, pp. 15–32.

11　UNICEF (2018) 'Guest blog: The impact of labour interventions on breastfeeding and infant health'. *Baby Friendly Initiative*. Available at: www.unicef.org.uk/babyfriendly/impact-of-labour-interventions/

12　*Biological Nurturing Home* (2019). Available at: www.biologicalnurturing.com/ (Accessed: 12 July 2021).

13　Colson, S. (2019). *Biological Nurturing: Instinctual Breastfeeding*. London: Pinter & Martin. Available at: www.pinterandmartin.com/biological-nurturing

14　Baby Buddy App: (2021) Pregnancy, birth and baby support: Best Beginnings. https://play. google.com/store/apps/details?id=uk.org.bestbeginnings.babybuddy&hl=en_GB&gl=US

15　Ibid.

16　McAndrew, F. *et al.* (2012) 'Infant Feeding Survey 2010', p. 186. Available at: https://sp.ukdataservice.ac.uk/doc/7281/mrdoc/pdf/7281_ifs-uk-2010_report.pdf

6   Some breastfeeding challenges

Many women in the UK experience early challenges with breastfeeding after birth and unfortunately may stop earlier than they intended, but with appropriate support could have been enabled to continue. Some babies are sleepy for the first few days and their mothers may have problems with positioning and attaching them; parents may worry that they are not making enough colostrum or breastmilk; mothers may have anatomical concerns, such as the size of their breasts, flat or long nipples; and may have emotional issues, such as aversion or anxiety and depression. They may worry about their babies being unable to breastfeed because of tongue tie or having other structural issues. Social media may have played a part in increasing some of these concerns, so parents may have picked up on unsubstantiated information. Most of the practical problems that parents face when starting to breastfeed are surmountable with appropriate support from trained midwives and health visitors, but specialist support should be available for the more complex issues.

In this chapter I will look at the common reasons why so many women stop breastfeeding in the early days and weeks after birth and how we can support them through these situations. I will also cover some of the more complex physical and emotional problems.

What are the early challenges parents may face with breastfeeding?

Infant feeding surveys have shown us how more women in the UK are starting to breastfeed since the 1970s, although exclusive breastfeeding at 6 months in 2010 was the lowest rate in the world.[1] There are encouraging signs from a Scottish survey in 2019[2] which showed that, through their national investment in training staff to support mothers, there was rise of exclusive breastfeeding at the health visitor's 6–8 week contact from 44% to 53% in those mothers who had started breastfeeding after birth.

What did the last infant feeding survey in 2010 tell us about the difficulties?

The Infant Feeding Survey reported[3] that mothers found the following difficulties in the first week after birth:

- the baby was not sucking/rejecting the breast (33%)
- mothers had painful breasts (22%)
- mothers felt that they have insufficient milk (17%).

In the second week mothers said:

- they thought they had insufficient milk (28%)
- the baby was 'too demanding' or 'always hungry' (17%)

DOI: 10.4324/9781003139775-6

- the baby was not sucking/rejecting the breast (22%)
- they had painful breasts or nipples (21%).

Why do some new-born babies not want to breastfeed after birth?

So many women experience their babies not wanting to suck or 'reject' the breasts in the first two weeks after birth (33% and 22% respectively). There must be other reasons for this occurring in the early postnatal period, such as drugs used in labour.

Breastfeeding should be seen as a continuum from birth, or the fourth trimester of pregnancy. As discussed in the last chapter, babies are hard-wired with strong instincts to crawl up their mothers' bodies and find the breasts for themselves and latch on, especially when in skin-to-skin contact with the mother. A mother's areola usually darkens in pregnancy which may help to guide the baby to the breast, as does the sebum secreted by the raised bumps on them called Montgomery glands, the smell of which appears to attract babies to the breasts. Artificial oxytocin (syntocinon) is often used to accelerate labour and there is some evidence that it interferes with the mother's production of natural oxytocin. Fentanyl is used for epidural anaesthesia and pethidine (an analgesic) can cross the placenta and may make infants sleepy. Evidence for how babies can be affected by these drugs is unclear and controversial but there is no doubt that at present many babies in the UK are very sleepy after birth.

Parents should be prepared for the possibility that their new-born infants can be very sleepy. If they have expressed frozen colostrum from 36 weeks of pregnancy, this can be defrosted and given to their babies if they do not attach to their breasts after birth, which will avoid the use of artificial milk. In this way their babies' gut flora and immunity can be protected and mothers' milk supplies continue to be stimulated. Mothers will need to continue with hand expressing and feeding it to their babies in syringes.

This first week of their baby's life is a difficult time for parents emotionally as well as physically, as they adjust to caring for their new arrival. They are confused and concerned about their baby's well-being, because they were given information in pregnancy about the benefits of breastfeeding and expected help from midwives and doctors, but too frequently they may be told to give their baby formula. The sad result is that this may lead to some of them giving up breastfeeding completely, despite really wanting to continue.

Trained healthcare staff or peer support should be available on the wards, to facilitate skin-to-skin contact, and support mothers to build up their milk supplies. They can observe them positioning and attaching their babies to their breasts encouraging effective feeding, as described in the last chapter. This should avoid another common problem which is painful nipples (22% and 21% respectively), allowing comfortable breastfeeding and following their feeding intentions.

Working on a hospital postnatal ward, I was very surprised how sleepy the babies were after birth. I found that sometimes on their first day they were so deeply asleep it was almost impossible to wake them for feeding. Often mothers were supported to start hand-expressing colostrum and to feed it to them with a syringe. Sometimes this had the effect of waking them enough, so they could then latch on the breasts. The more confident mothers were able to do this, especially those who had learnt to hand-express colostrum before the birth, but others were discouraged from trying again because of the small volume of colostrum, or they thought their babies just did not like their breasts. Unfortunately, some were advised by health professionals to give bottles of formula, rather than continue with expressing colostrum and giving it with a syringe:

- which had the effect of stretching their stomachs with larger volumes of formula, coming with a faster flow, so the babies were not satisfied with smaller volumes of colostrum.
- some babies were confused by the different sucking action on a bottle teat and had even more problems latching when offered the breast.
- also, the formula had a negative effect on the baby's microbiome which could have a long-term health impact. It really helped when mothers brought expressed colostrum with them into hospital, because their babies were able to have this from syringes which avoided these problems.

Why does skin-to-skin help babies latch on the breasts?

I discussed skin-to-skin after birth in the last chapter, but it can also be helpful if babies are struggling to latch on the breasts in the first few weeks after birth. Mothers can be encouraged to keep their babies there for as long as possible, to encourage their natural instincts to find the breasts and latch on themselves. Laid back positions, with babies lying on top of mothers' bodies, can help them take the lead by feeling the mothers' skin with their cheeks and begin 'rooting' by turning their heads from side to side opening their mouths very wide. It is also a wonderful way of having a close cuddle and both of their bodies and brains relating to each other. This leads to long-term relationships and can protect their mental health which will be considered in the next chapter.

Is it normal for nipples to become sore when starting breastfeeding?

Many people assume that breastfeeding will be painful, and 22% of mothers in the first week and 21% in the second week reported this as a problem in 2010.

Sensitivity of the nipples in the first week after birth is common, but this should only last for the first 20 seconds or less at the beginning of the feed, as the baby draws the nipple into the back of her mouth. Any pain or sensitivity which lasts longer than this is a sign that the baby is not latched effectively and the mother's nipple is likely to be a different shape when the baby comes off the breast than it was before the feed. This indicates that the nipple is rubbing on the baby's hard palate at the front of the mouth and may be flattened by this to make it 'lipstick shaped' – a sign of poor attachment. This mother will require urgent help with positioning and attaching her baby, and a full feeding assessment from a trained person is required to ensure the baby receives a good flow of milk and breastfeeding becomes comfortable. Once she has mastered this skill, she will ensure that her baby grows well, breastfeeding is comfortable and she can avoid other problems associated with poor milk transfer. These tips may be helpful when you are supporting mothers to encourage babies to open their mouths wider and achieve a deeper, comfortable latch for them (see Figure 6.1 and 6.2).

Why do some parents worry that they have insufficient milk?

I have mentioned this problem about concerns about the volumes of breastmilk and colostrum several times in this book. Society doubts that women's bodies will produce

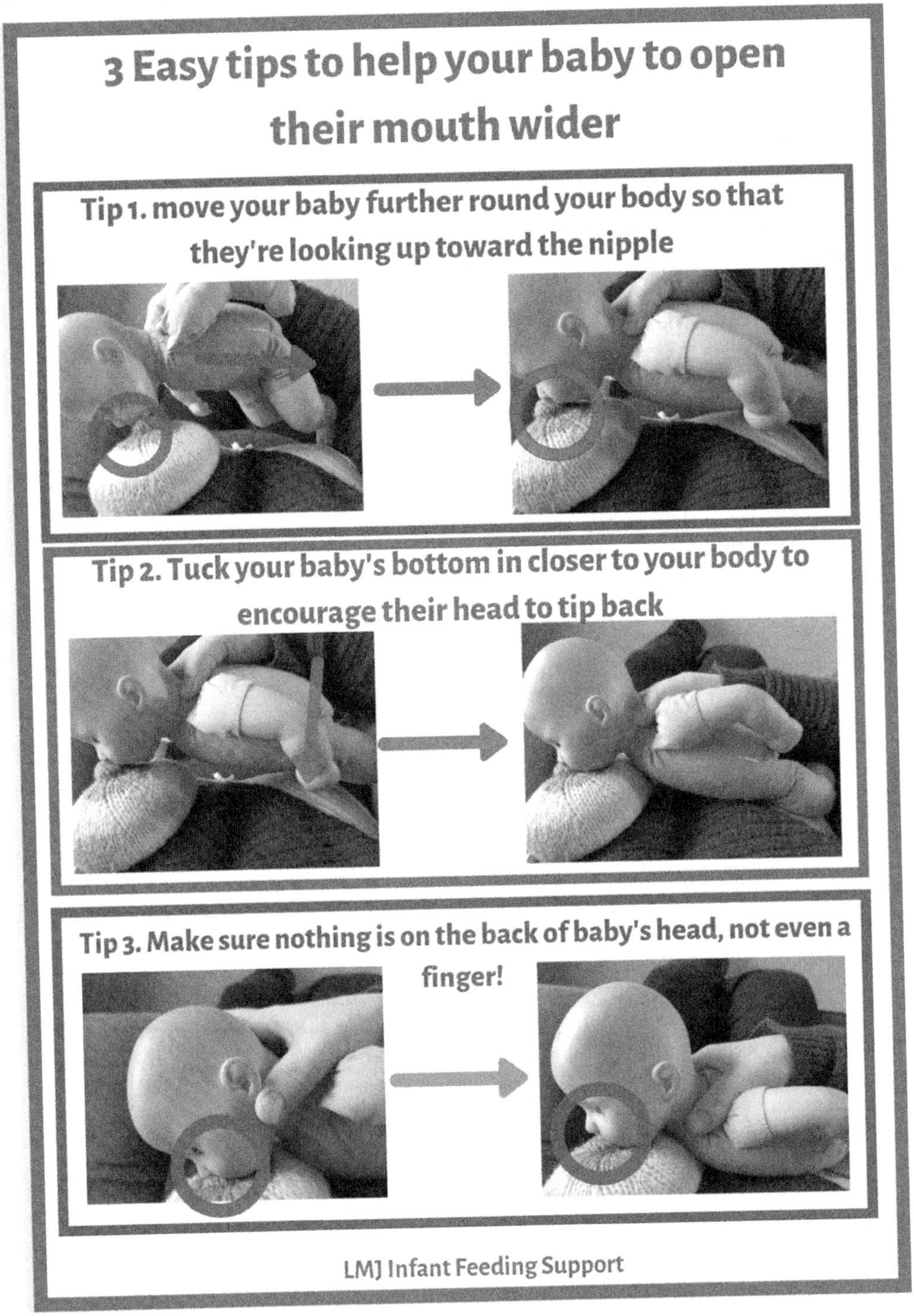

3 Easy tips to help your baby to open their mouth wider

Tip 1. move your baby further round your body so that they're looking up toward the nipple

Tip 2. Tuck your baby's bottom in closer to your body to encourage their head to tip back

Tip 3. Make sure nothing is on the back of baby's head, not even a finger!

LMJ Infant Feeding Support

Figure 6.1 Tips to encourage babies to open their mouths
Source: Courtesy of Lucy Webber IBCLC

Thumbs up!
for a deeper latch

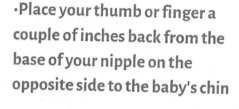

This quick, easy tip can make a world of difference

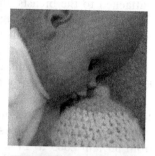

·Start position

·Place your thumb or finger a couple of inches back from the base of your nipple on the opposite side to the baby's chin

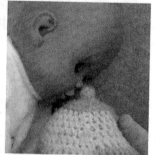

·Pull your thumb backward or push into the breast tissue. This will form a bulge on the other side of the breast.
·Keep the bottom lip in the same spot now.
·When baby opens wide, bring them swiftly forward, chin leading.
·At the same time nudge your thumb/finger slightly forward. The bulge you created will roll onto their tongue and nipple to the back of their mouth.
·Now admire your nice deep latch!

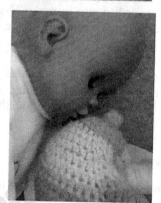

☆ The bottom lip needs to start, and stay, well away from the base of the nipple no matter what technique you're using ☆

LMJ Infant Feeding Support

Figure 6.2 Tips for a deeper latch
Source: Courtesy of Lucy Webber IBCLC

enough to sustain babies. We cannot see how much babies are taking from the breasts and when women express colostrum there are only small volumes. Babies' stomachs are small and 5–10ml of colostrum is sufficient for their needs and contentment.

The main reasons given in 2010 for stopping in the second week were similar to the first week, with the addition that the baby is 'too demanding' or 'always hungry', which may be due to parents' expectations which may be for regular time intervals between feeds rather than the frequent feeds of most exclusively breastfed babies in the early weeks. It could also be that when babies are poorly attached to the breasts, the transfer of milk may not be efficient and mothers may think they do not have enough milk. Parents can monitor their babies' urine and stool output which will give them confidence that their babies are feeding well.

However, the good news is that the proportion of mothers citing insufficient milk as a reason for stopping breastfeeding decreased between 2005 and 2010, particularly at one week from 42% to 28%. This may indicate an increase in parents' knowledge about milk supply and how it builds up in the early weeks to meet babies' needs. The other encouraging sign at this time was that the proportion of mothers who stopped breast-feeding as a result of painful breasts or nipples reduced from 30% in 2005 to 21% in 2010. This suggests parents are receiving better support in positioning and attaching their babies and understanding breastmilk production, as more midwives and health visitors are trained to UNICEF Baby Friendly standards.

Do parents understand new-born behaviour?

Many new parents may interpret their babies as being hungry and demanding and think the reason for this is because they are not taking enough colostrum/milk from the breasts. Images on TV of babies happily formula feeding and sleeping contentedly are frequently seen in advertisements for follow-on formula milk, suggesting that breast-milk is not satisfying and if they want a night's sleep, they need to give formula. Most new-borns want to breastfeed frequently in the first week, which stimulates mothers' milk supply, so we need to give reassurance that this does not suggest a problem. Babies love to have close contact, especially in skin-to-skin with their parents, hearing the familiar noises of their voices, heartbeat, breathing and tummy rumbles! This helps to build relationships, improves babies' emotional brain development and feelings of trust. Oxytocin is secreted by both parents and babies when they are close, and this helps with breastmilk production and let down.

Why do some mothers get painful or cracked nipples?

When you see a mother experiencing pain at your new-baby visit, you can encourage her to take the baby off the breast, by slipping her finger into the corner of her mouth to break the suction, and then show her how to *re-position her baby*. You can demonstrate this to her with a doll and knitted breast, following the acronym CHIN as described in Chapter 5.

Then she can *attach her baby* by bringing her to the breast, nose level with her nipple, with her mouth open wide, her head tilted back and her chin leading with the mother's nipple aimed to the baby's top lip. As she brings her swiftly to the breast, with a wide-open mouth (like a yawn), she will achieve an *asymmetrical latch* which is characterised by more of the areola being seen over her top lip than below her bottom one (Figure 6.3).

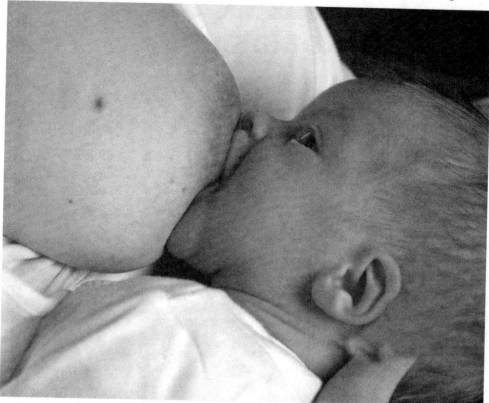

Figure 6.3 Baby well attached on the breast
Source: Images supplied by Real Baby Milk, a project of Pollen CIC.

Small adjustments can make a big difference!

If the feed continues to be painful, then you can support her with re-attaching her baby, if you feel confident to do so and have received training to UNICEF Baby Friendly Standards. The koala position (Figure 6.4) and the laid-back position (Figure 6.5) can help improve the baby's attachment.

If you do not feel confident in these practical skills, ask an experienced colleague, or refer the mother to your local infant feeding team, breastfeeding counsellor or lactation consultant (IBCLC).

Do creams help sore and cracked nipples?

Mothers often apply nipple creams which will help with healing sore or cracked nipples. However, the Montgomery glands in the areola make a perfect, protective serum which lubricates their nipples, and contains an antiseptic property. These little glands become more obvious and active in pregnancy and appear as small, raised bumps in the areola tissue. You can suggest to mothers that they avoid any creams, or even shower gels on the breasts to preserve this special fluid, to retain the natural smell of the breasts, which babies love.

After feeds mothers can express a small amount of colostrum or milk on their nipples and gently spread it with a fingertip and then air-dry. Some mothers may decide to use a

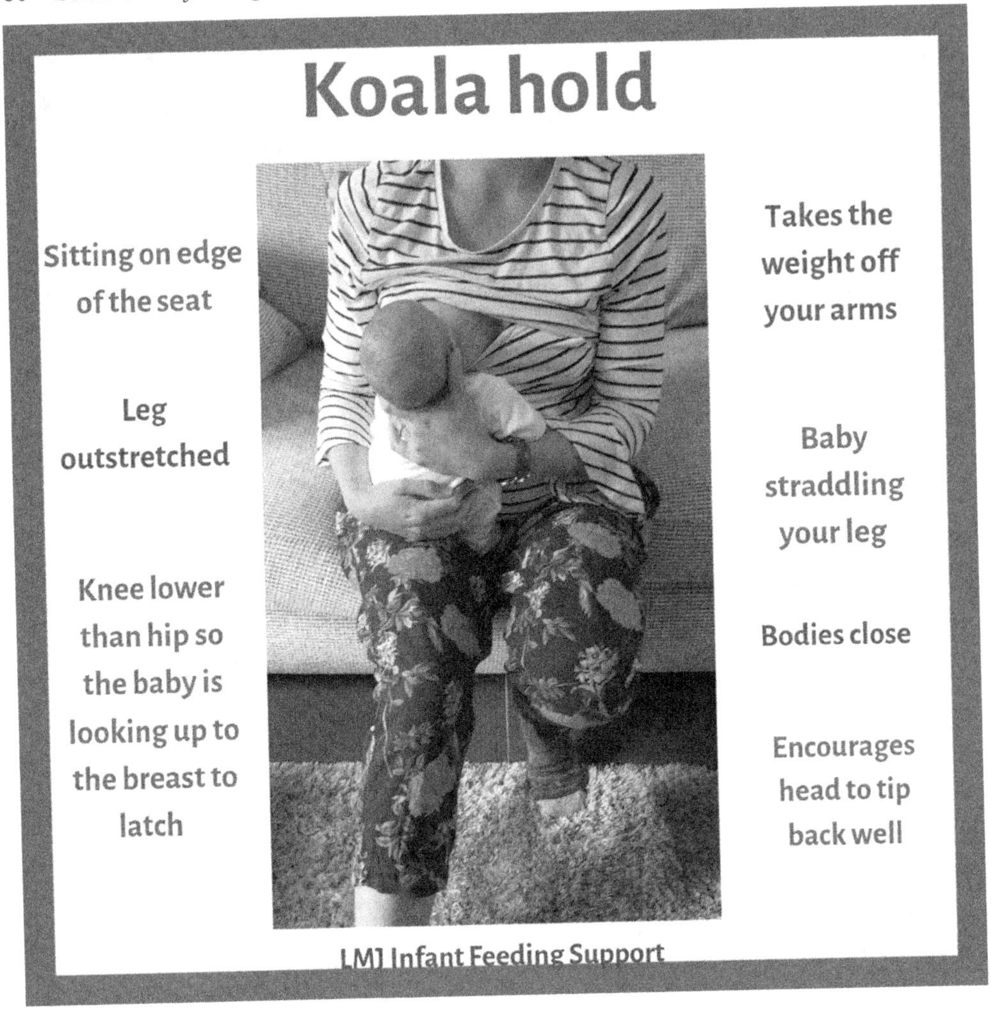

Koala hold

Sitting on edge of the seat

Leg outstretched

Knee lower than hip so the baby is looking up to the breast to latch

Takes the weight off your arms

Baby straddling your leg

Bodies close

Encourages head to tip back well

LMJ Infant Feeding Support

Figure 6.4 Koala position for a deeper latch
Source: Courtesy of Lucy Webber IBCLC

lanolin cream, or gel-net gauze to help very damaged nipples heal and stop them sticking to breast pads or bras and find this helps with healing. These creams will not work on their own without improvement to positioning and attaching their babies and some mothers may be sensitive to lanolin, but if mothers decide to use them, they need to do so with care.

What are other common problems mothers may face in the early weeks of breastfeeding?

Concerns about nipple shape and size – many women worry that their nipples may present problems and they may not be suitable for breastfeeding. Babies do not know that there are different sizes and shapes of breasts and nipples, they only know their mothers'!

Babies can latch on flat and inverted nipples, but mothers may need extra support at the beginning with holding and latching their babies. Babies need to be positioned with

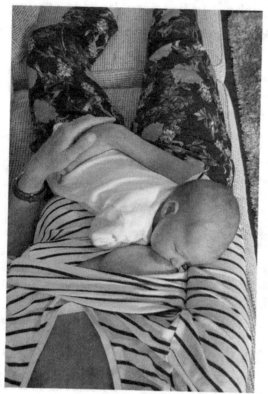

Laid Back Breastfeeding

Less nipple pain and damage than in parent led latching

Comfortable and relaxing

Both bodies fully supported

Give it a try

LMJ Infant Feeding Support

Figure 6.5 Laid-back position to reduce nipple pain
Source: Courtesy of Lucy Webber IBCLC

their noses aligned with the nipples. The 'exaggerated latch' can often help. Here mothers hold their breasts, making a C-shape with their hands, cupping the breasts but not moving their natural position. They can then apply gentle pressure using their thumbs on the areola next to the baby's top lip, so tilting their nipple upwards towards the top of the baby's mouth. The baby can then be brought to the breast, leading with their chin and taking the lower areola into their mouth and the nipple can then unfold to touch the roof of their mouth (see Figure 6.6). The pressure on the areola needs to be maintained until the baby has drawn the nipple far back in their mouth, resting on the margin with the soft palate and they start drawing the milk. This is also known as the 'flipple', so called because the mother tilts an upturned nipple away from her baby. The nipple is 'flicked' to the back of the baby's mouth at the exact moment when the bottom lip and chin connect with the underside of the areola. See the video on YouTube.[4]

Breast shaping

Good for small mouths, big breasts, babies struggling to latch, as it makes the breast more mouth shaped

'C' hold   'U' hold

@KathrynStaggIBCLC

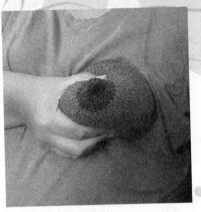
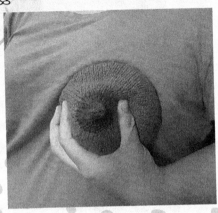

Use with rugby/
football hold

Use with cross
cradle hold

Figure 6.6 Breast shaping can help
Source: Courtesy of Kathryn Stagg IBCLC

Long nipples can be more challenging because babies' mouths may not be big enough to draw the whole nipple far enough back which may mean the sides of the nipples rub on the hard palate and become misshapen and painful, babies may gag and struggle to transfer milk effectively. Specialist support may be needed to optimise their positioning and attachment, so babies can breastfeed more easily. Sometimes mothers may need to express their milk to give to their babies in addition to breastfeeding which will also maintain their milk supplies. The good news here is that babies' mouths grow so breastfeeding becomes easier over time!

Engorgement can occur in the first week after birth as the supply adjusts to needs. Mothers can experience painful, hard, hot shiny breasts, due to tissue swelling which makes it hard for babies to latch on. This is due to the increased blood supply to the breasts 3–4 days after birth, as they fill up with transitional milk. Today babies are usually fed responsively which keeps the breasts softer. A supportive bra with adjustable hooks will help keep them feeling more comfortable. Mothers could try some warm compresses with gentle stroking from the nipples backwards to move some of the oedema (swelling) away from the nipples before breastfeeding. Some mothers also find that milk will leak out to soften the breasts if they have a warm bath or shower before feeding. They can also encourage this by gentle massage or hand expressing. After feeds they can apply cold compresses or cold Savoy cabbage leaves inside their bras, for 20 minutes after feeds, three times a day, which can reduce heat and inflammation, which will be soothing. Anti-inflammatory drugs may relieve some of the discomfort and lower any fever caused by the inflammation. Mothers can be reassured that this is a temporary problem and after a few days their breasts will be softer and the 'supply and demand' will mean they will just make milk for one baby.

Blocked ducts can occur when they get blocked by thick fatty milk, causing a lumpy, very tender segment of the breast which is usually discoloured. Any mother suffering from these symptoms should have a whole feed assessed by an infant feeding specialist, breast-feeding counsellor, or a lactation consultant, who will be able to help the mother improve her baby's attachment and suggest ways of clearing the duct before it deteriorates into mastitis or breast abscess. It is a plumbing problem and the baby is best at clearing it! It may have been caused by the baby not being attached well and not draining the breast effectively, or by outside pressure such as a hand, bra, clothing or sling pressing on the breast. The mother could try changing her feeding position and aiming the baby's chin over the blocked area, or diagonally opposite it. Some mothers have found that if they lie their babies on a flat surface and they go into an 'all fours' position over them to breast-feed, gravity can help the babies draw out the blockage below them and help to drain the breast. Mothers may want to ask their partners to help with this position.

Hand-expressing after feeds or while in a bath or shower can help to drain the duct, especially if she is able to position her thumbs or fingers over the blocked area. Also, the mother can stroke the affected area in a shower or bath with a wide-toothed comb, after applying a small amount of oil over the affected area, which can also help to move the blockage. Some mothers do seem to have frequent blocked ducts and need to be vigilant at checking their breasts every day in the shower; massaging or using an electric toothbrush over any lumpy areas may help with the drainage. Some have found that reducing the fat content in their diet helps.

Mastitis may follow on from an uncleared blocked duct because milk stasis is an ideal breeding ground for bacteria. Here her breast becomes very painful and an area becomes hard, hot and inflamed and she is likely to develop a fever. She can become generally very unwell, feeling as if she has 'flu and can take over-the-counter analgesics (you could look at the evidence-based drugs in the Drugs in Breastmilk section on the Breastfeeding Network website).[5] If the mother is unable to clear the inflamed segment of her breast within 12–24 hours she will need to consult her GP, who is likely to pre-scribe antibiotics, but while she takes them she still needs to continue to try to clear the breast to prevent abscess formation, and take probiotics to prevent possible thrush infection. She will need support from her partner and family at this difficult time because she is likely to be feeling very unwell for a few days. Infectious mastitis used to spread around maternity units but rarely happens now. NICE has recently published a guideline on mastitis and breast abscess and states that accumulated milk in the breast causes an inflammatory response which may or may not progress to infection. The most common organism associated with infective mastitis is Staphylcoccus aureus.[6]

Breast abscesses may develop after infective mastitis when a collection of pus seals itself off, and antibiotics penetrate poorly. The breast develops a lump and the skin over it is often discoloured or has a pitted appearance like 'orange peel' and diagnosis is made by ultrasound scan. The only effective treatment is by medical intervention to aspirate it with a needle, guided by an ultrasound scan. Usually, several aspirations are needed until the abscess has disappeared completely. This treatment is preferable and less invasive than open surgery to remove it leaving an open wound, which has to be packed with gauze, so that it heals from the inside outwards, and feeding from that breast becomes very difficult. The preferred treatment is aspiration without an open wound, so breastfeeding from the affected breast can continue.

Galactoceles are also lumps in the breast which can occur after blocked ducts have sealed themselves off as cysts but contain fluid or milk rather than pus. It is important to investigate any lumps in the breast by ultrasound to confirm the diagnosis and ensure there is no malignancy.

Why is it important to offer both breasts at each feed?

Babies follow their hunger feelings and will finish feeding from the first breast when their tummies feel full. They may come off decisively by pulling their heads back and spitting out the breast and sometimes look full and 'milk drunk', or they may stop sucking and fall asleep. Commonly, after a short period of time, often 10–15 minutes, they start showing feeding cues again indicating they want more from the second breast but sometimes they indicate they have taken enough from the first side. They will decide how much they will take from the second breast and will often feed for a much shorter period of time here. The research on foremilk and hindmilk has been misunderstood and some health professionals have given wrong advice about this. Babies take what their bodies need from the breasts and understand how to get it! We need to follow their lead and the book *Baby-led Breastfeeding* describes this process.[7] Are there other causes of sore nipples? The most common cause of nipple pain is poor positioning and attachment of the baby's mouth on the breast, but it can occur in other conditions such as tongue tie, thrush and Raynaud's syndrome.

Tongue tie is a condition where the skin under the baby's tongue, the lingual frenulum, is short, making the tongue heart-shaped in anterior tongue tie, which can affect tongue movement, making it difficult for her to latch on the breast, especially when it is associated with high palates. It can run in families and boys are more likely to be affected than girls. After breastfeeds the mother's nipples may look pinched and 'lipstick' shaped and can be extremely painful.

Not all babies with visible tight anterior tongue ties have problems breastfeeding. There is a lack of good quality evidence on tongue tie, but a full feeding history and assessment of tongue movement as well as an observation of a breastfeed needs to be done, before a diagnosis can be made. Some visible frenula are stretchy and elastic and can move to draw the nipples to the back of their mouths without any problem. Tight anterior or posterior frenula can cause painful nipples or blocked ducts and some babies may struggle to obtain good milk transfer because their tongues cannot move adequately to draw their mothers' nipples to the back of their mouths.

When assessing tongue movement, we need to consider the way it extends, elevates and moves sideways. It is also worthwhile to consider palate shape and how the back of the tongue moves when we consider suckling ability and seal formation. This should be done by a breastfeeding specialist or lactation consultant observing a whole breastfeed.

Parents are often very anxious about their baby having a tongue tie, because today it is commonly talked about on social media and they may be concerned about how their babies' speech will develop if they do not have a tongue tie release performed.

A lactation consultant and infant feeding lead, Julie Peris told me of her experience of supporting parents with babies with tongue tie:

> In my experience parents need reassurance and support with latching much more often than they need a referral to a tongue tie practitioner. Even if a baby is found to have a genuine degree of tongue tie which restricts function some parents reasonably choose not to have the frenulum cut. They may hope that the frenulum stretches over time improving tongue function (and this often does happen) or they may decide that the risk of a wound under baby's tongue and the resulting pain may complicate breastfeeding more than the restrictive frenulum does.
>
> When a baby has a posterior tongue tie the frenulum may be very short and right at the back of the tongue and only visible to someone who really inspects the underside of the tongue. However, this frenulum may be tough and sinewy and really prevent the tongue moving well.

How can we assess for tongue tie?

This should usually be carried out by a lactation consultant in tongue tie because it is important to get the correct diagnosis and Julie Peris told me the following:

> In order to make a valid assessment of whether a baby has a tongue tie we need to think about how well the tongue moves and what the tongue function is like, rather than the appearance of the frenulum.
>
> When your gloved finger is in the baby's mouth and up against the hard palate it will trigger the suckling reflex. You should feel the baby's tongue suckling against your finger in a wave like motion originating from the back and rippling through to the tip. Some babies initially appear to have restrictive tongue function but upon doing this you may feel how well the back of the tongue moves and lifts as it suckles against your finger and forms a seal around your finger.
>
> When assessing tongue function we need to consider three main areas:
>
> The best way to assess tongue extension is to place a gloved finger on the centre of the baby's lower lip. She will automatically try to extend her tongue to at least past her lower gum and ideally to the finger on the lower lip. Once the baby has extended her tongue, you can assess lateralisation by slowly sliding your finger along to the corners of the mouth. Most babies won't follow your finger neatly, but the baby should have some sideways movement of the tongue. You might see the edges along one side of the tongue lift. If the baby is sliding her tongue to the left side of her mouth you might see some movement on the right side of her tongue.
>
> Finally, you can assess Elevation by seeing how well the baby's tongue lifts in the mouth. It is easiest to assess this when she is crying. The ability of the tongue to elevate is more important than extension and lateralisation. We hope that the baby's tongue will lift by at least a third of the available height in their mouth.
>
> It is worth bearing in mind that some babies do not have a restrictive frenulum but will present with difficulties moving their tongue in the ways described above perhaps because of residual birth trauma. Taking a full history is therefore obviously of vital importance when supporting breastfeeding mothers.
>
> A small minority of babies may have such restrictive tongue function that a frenulotomy is genuinely needed before they breastfeed effectively or even efficient

bottle feeding is possible. These babies will have great difficulty latching even with optimal support, or they may manage to latch, but not well. These babies may not be able to maintain a groove around the nipple and may click during a feed as their tongue repeatedly releases its seal. Feeding is inefficient. The baby may need frequent long feeds and as with other cases of sub-optimal latch may be unsettled with digestive pain because they are unable to maintain the feed long enough to access the fatty dense milk and may receive only high lactose (milk sugar) milk. Mother may develop very sore nipples. They will need emotional support as well as support to protect their milk supply while waiting for a frenulotomy.

For this small minority of babies a tongue tie release will really help them in the long term, but in the short term immediately after the tongue tie release things may not seem to significantly improve. The baby may be orally averse after having the intrusion of scissors to snip their frenulum and the tongue may now be very loose and mobile. Baby will have to learn how to move their tongue in a wave like milking motion at the breast after the tongue has been anchored down to the floor of the mouth. These families need ongoing long-term support.

For tongue tie that does not require surgery, you could suggest the mother tries to use 'the exaggerated latch' when latching her baby.[8]

In order to meet the needs of all families it is important that we are able to support them with optimal attachment and positioning, listen to their concerns in a mother-centred approach, reassure and help them understand the basics of tongue function. This understanding will help avoid unnecessary diagnosis, oral surgery and angst while protecting breastfeeding and appropriate referral for those small number of babies with genuine restrictive tongue function.

Thrush caused by the fungus Candida Albicans used to be thought to be a very common cause of sore nipples, but many mothers found that if they improved their babies' positioning and attachment on their breasts, their pain disappeared. Thrush is a yeast which lives on our skins and can colonise any broken skin in our bodies, and nipples and babies' mouths can be affected too. It will affect both breasts and can cause severe shooting pains after feeds, but it is important to diagnose it before any treatment is prescribed, by referring to a GP for a swab of the nipples. There may be blanching or peeling of the skin over the areolar tissue and you might see white plaques on the inside of babies' mouths (white tongues on their own are not necessarily signs). If the swabs indeed come back positive for thrush, then mothers and babies need to be treated at the same time. The mothers can be prescribed anti-fungal creams for their nipples and oral drops for babies' mouths, which they can apply after feeds. Sometimes mothers can report diffuse, systemic thrush with skin rashes and painful mouths or throats and will need oral anti-fungal treatment. Self-help measures can prevent cross-infection from mothers to babies by regular hand washing and using a different towel from others in the household; taking probiotic tablets or acidophilus capsules can help and some mothers also find reducing sugars and yeasts in their diets also helps. The Breastfeeding Network's (BfN) website has some very useful information on diagnosis and treatment.[9]

Raynaud's syndrome[10] – mothers are more likely to experience vasospasm in their nipples if they already suffer from it in their fingers and toes. This can cause severe, deep, stabbing, pain after feeds with both nipples being affected and they become blanched (or sometimes blue). You can refer the mother to her GP for a full assessment and sometimes a drug called nifedipine will be prescribed, which has the effect of encouraging vaso-dilation to relieve her symptoms. Simple remedies such as heat or wheat pads can help. You can ensure that she is positioning and attaching her baby well, especially if the nipples also look squashed after feeds.

Is eczema on the nipples a problem?

Women who have eczema may find they experience itching of the nipples which can result in damage. It is worth avoiding any irritants such as nipple creams, shower gels or even deodorants near the breasts. They can apply their emollient creams regularly which should reduce the itching, dryness and thickened skin areas.[11]

Are there other maternal medical conditions that might affect breastfeeding?

Polycystic Ovary Syndrome (PCOS) – some women with PCOS may experience problems establishing an adequate milk supply for their babies. Their breasts may be 'tubular' shaped and may not respond to pregnancy hormones, so mothers may not notice changes in their breasts, such as an increase in size and darker areola pigment development. Skin-to-skin with their babies helps breastfeeding hormone levels rise, as well as frequent breastfeeding and expressing which can help to build prolactin levels and milk supply. A few women find that despite this they need to supplement their babies with formula after breastfeeds. They may have worked really hard to stimulate their supplies and need reassurance that their babies will benefit from the close contact they are receiving and any amount of breastmilk.

Why do parents frequently worry about their babies having reflux?

Posseting in babies is very common, when a baby brings up some milk after a feed or vomits small quantities during or just after feeding. It is usually caused by immaturity of the digestive system and poor sphincter tone at the top of the stomach which improves as baby grows and becomes more upright. Small vomits or regurgitation of mouthfuls of milk means that the baby's clothes have to be changed frequently and babies ask to be fed again. It usually starts before 8 weeks of age, as babies begin to take larger volumes of milk, and often stops once babies reach 8–12 months.

In a few cases reflux can cause babies a lot of pain when acid travels up the oesophagus and is known as gastro-oesophageal reflux disease (GORD). This can lead to babies becoming very distressed, having abdominal pain and spitting up a lot of milk. Some parents believe that their babies have 'silent reflux' but there are no obvious signs because the baby does not bring up milk. Many parents worry that their babies may be suffering from this when they are very unsettled, their abdomens feel hard and they may not be gaining weight as expected. Babies who are breastfed may benefit by improving their positioning and attachment on the breasts. I mentioned earlier that if babies are not latching well, they may be receiving large volumes of foremilk, which contains high levels of lactose and this may be causing a degree of lactose intolerance.

Once the latch is better, the baby takes a lower volume feed, with higher fat content, and lower lactose and in my experience, the abdominal discomfort reduces, babies become more settled and gain weight better. Formula companies have designed 'special medical conditions' formulae for babies suffering from reflux and some parents feel they should try this rather than improving their breastfeeding techniques, but babies will then lose much of the benefits of breastmilk. Research into these milks has been limited and the controls over their marketing to health professionals not controlled. Some babies are given medication by GPs and paediatricians rather than mothers given specialist breastfeeding help with their positioning and attachment.

How can we support mothers with physical or mental health issues that may cause problems with breastfeeding?

Mothers may have physical disabilities and require additional help from partners and families and may ask you for extra support with breastfeeding. They may need adaptations to their homes or equipment to enable them to position their babies. They may also seek reassurances from you that breastfeeding is possible which may be easier for them than having to prepare formula feeds and sterilise bottles and teats.

When a mother has other chronic medical conditions and has to take regular medication, it is important for her to check with her GP that these are suitable for breastfeeding. The BfN website[12] and the LactMed App[13] have very useful information on drugs and breastfeeding, so you could direct her to this, or find out information for her.

Mental health illness during the perinatal period is very common, but if mothers receive enough support, they can have positive experiences of breastfeeding, which can help to protect their moods and build their relationships with their babies. This will be discussed in full in Chapter 7, but here we will look at why some mothers may experience breastfeeding aversion and agitation.

Do we understand why some mothers get negative feelings and aversion when breastfeeding?

Zainab Yate has researched this subject and written a book called *When Breastfeeding Sucks: What You Need to Know about Breastfeeding Aversion and Agitation*, which concerns the negative feelings a few women may experience at some point in their breastfeeding journeys. She has explained some of her findings here:

> A small number of mothers can experience negative embodied emotions when breastfeeding.[14] These can include the medical condition of Dysphoric feelings (the opposite of euphoric, or a profound sense of unease), Milk Ejection Reflex (D-MER),[15] and the phenomenon of Breastfeeding Aversion and Agitation (Aversion).[16] As many of the mothers present with symptoms that may seem similar to post-natal depression or postnatal mood disorders at first glance, it is common for there to be misdiagnosis of these conditions in breastfeeding mothers. Consequently, incorrect treatments such as the prescription of SSRI anti-depressants can follow, which often do not alleviate the symptoms mothers struggle with. Mothers can experience both conditions as they are not mutually exclusive, and they are able to differentiate symptoms and onset of each experience when asked. It is useful for health visitors to understand these conditions as part of a differential diagnosis in order to appropriately refer mothers, and we can start by looking at D-MER.
>
> D-MER is characterised by a sudden onset of dysphoric feelings lasting less than 10 minutes at the beginning of a feed, with the most common negative emotions of

feeling tearful, irritable, panicky, oversensitive and sad, and has a significant pre-valence rate.[17] D-MER is hypothesised to occur due to two possible mechanisms, the first is a sudden drop in dopamine during the let-down,[18] the second an upre-gulation of the stress response due to negative pairing of oxytocin during the let-down.[19] The onset of this condition is often from birth and can self-correct by 9 months, however this differs greatly from mother to mother, depending on the severity of the symptoms and her access to a support network in order to manage the condition and continue breastfeeding. There is little known about risk factors, aside from that mothers who experience D-MER will often go on to experience it with subsequent breastfeeding journeys. There is also very little evidenced-based literature that shows what can help, although management through diet seems a common approach by lactation clinicians, as well as use of particular supplements. Moberg and Tackett also propose that Cognitive Behavioural Therapies (CBT) and Mindfulness interventions will help.

Aversion, on the other hand, is characterised by distinct negative emotions of anger and agitation, a skin-crawling or itching sensation and an over-whelming urge to de-latch the baby or child.[20] The onset, duration and severity vary from dyad to dyad – depending on the underlying cause for experiencing the phenom-enon. The majority of mothers want support to help manage their aversion as they desire to continue breastfeeding. The prevalence of aversion is not yet known; however, it is known that the following cohorts commonly experience aversion; those who are breastfeeding through persistent pain and discomfort, those who are tandem feeding or breastfeeding through pregnancy, those who have sensory sen-sitivities or are on the autism spectrum, and those who are survivors of sexual abuse or childhood trauma. Using the step-by-step acronym 'BROMPHALICC' to identify triggers and appropriate interventions can help alleviate symptoms. These include: 1. Breastfeeding aversion triggers, 2. Reactionary behaviours, 3. Ovulation and Menstruation, 4. Prevention of escalation of the vicious cycle of aversion, 5. Hydration increase and nutritional improvement, 6. Active Distraction if the nursling is older than 12 months, 7. Lifestyle changes to make time and space for infant feeding and motherhood, 8 Interventional therapies including mindfulness, 9. Counselling for pain management or trauma, and 10. Cessation of breastfeeding with support.

Often, simply having the symptoms of negative emotions triggered by breast-feeding acknowledged and mothers becoming aware of the conditions can bring relief, and allow the mother to continue to breastfeed. Using alternative or com-plementary therapies to relax the mother, aid the milk ejection reflex and enhance the overall breastfeeding experience[21] to a more positive one can reduce symptoms. Many mothers also join peer to peer support groups, such as those on social media that can also help mothers to understand their experiences, their personal triggers and how to alleviate the symptoms.

Fear of disclosure often occurs, due both D-MER and Aversion not being well known about, and due to shame and guilt mothers have for feeling the negative emotions when breastfeeding. As a key starting point, mothers can be asked; 'how do you feel when breastfeeding?', to decipher if a mother is experiencing challenges with emotions when breastfeeding. Ideally, we would want to hear that the hor-mone oxytocin is having a positive and calming effect on the mother when the nursling is suckling. If a mother is predominately having negative emotions that are dysphoric in nature when breastfeeding, it may be that she has the condition of D-MER, especially if these are only within the first 10 minutes – coinciding with the milk ejection reflex. If she experiences negative emotions throughout a whole breastfeeding session, no matter how long it is, and the feelings are of anger and agitation, coupled with an urge to de-latch, she could be experiencing aversion. Either way, further investigation is likely required to rule out symptoms of negative emotions or mood changes are not due to other conditions such as postnatal depression or hyperthyroidism. In conclusion, it is important that a process of differential diagnosis is made so that you can refer the mother for appropriate assessment in order to prevent misdiagnosis, pharmacological treatment and interventions that are not efficacious – as well as the unwanted early cessation of breastfeeding which carries its own risks.

Breastfeeding challenges such as aversion can occur at any stage of a mother's breastfeeding journey, but they are more likely to occur in the first weeks after birth, as the baby adjusts to finding milk and extracting it from the breast and mother's supply adjusts to her needs.

In this chapter, I have also addressed some of the common physical and psychological challenges that mothers face. Many of the physical ones can be tackled by mothers receiving support from infant feeding leads, peer supporters or the more complex ones by breastfeeding counsellors or lactation consultants. The principles of effective positioning and attachment of the baby on the breast, as discussed in the previous chapter apply here too so that mothers can enjoy comfortable breastfeeding experiences.

Notes

1   Rollins, N. C. *et al.* (2016) 'Why invest, and what it will take to improve breastfeeding practices?', *The Lancet*, 387(10017), pp. 491–504.
2   'Infant Feeding Statistics Scotland' (2019) www.isdscotland.org/Health-Topics/Child-Health/Publications/2019-10-29/2019-10-29-Infant-Feeding-Report.pdf
3   McAndrew, F. *et al.* (2012) 'Infant Feeding Survey 2010'. Available at: https://sp.ukdataservice.ac.uk/doc/7281/mrdoc/pdf/7281_ifs-uk-2010_report.pdf
4   See www.youtube.com/watch?v=41fC0fQs1P8
5   The Breastfeeding Network (2021) 'Drugs in breastmilk – is it safe?'. Available at: www.breastfeedingnetwork.org.uk/detailed-information/drugs-in-breastmilk/
6   NICE (2021) *Mastitis and Breast Abscess.* Health topics A to Z – CKS. Available at: https://cks.nice.org.uk/topics/mastitis-breast-abscess/
7   Rapley, G. and Murkett, T. (2012) *Baby-led Breastfeeding.* London: Vermilion. Available at: www.penguin.co.uk/books/1085960/baby-led-breastfeeding/9780091935290
8   See www.youtube.com/watch?v=41fC0fQs1P8
9   The Breastfeeding Network (2021) 'Thrush (of the breast/nipple) and breastfeeding'. Available at: www.breastfeedingnetwork.org.uk/thrush-detailed/
10 The Breastfeeding Network (2021) 'Raynaud's phenomenon in breastfeeding mothers'. Available at: www.breastfeedingnetwork.org.uk/raynauds/
11 The Breastfeeding Network (2021) 'Eczema and breastfeeding'. Available at: www.breastfeedingnetwork.org.uk/eczema/
12 The Breastfeeding Network (2021) 'Drugs in breastmilk – is it safe?'. Available at: www.breastfeedingnetwork.org.uk/detailed-information/drugs-in-breastmilk/
13 National Library of Medicine (US) (2006) *Drugs and Lactation Database (LactMed).* www.ncbi.nlm.nih.gov/books/NBK501922/

14 Watkinson, M., Murray, C. and Simpson, J. (2016) 'Maternal experiences of embodied emotional sensations during breast feeding: An interpretative phenomenological analysis', *Midwifery*, 36, pp. 53–60.

15 Heise, A. M. and Wiessinger, D. (2011) 'Dysphoric milk ejection reflex: A case report', *International Breastfeeding Journal*, 6, p. 6.

16 Yate, Z. M. (2017) 'A qualitative study on negative emotions triggered by breastfeeding: Describing the phenomenon of breastfeeding/nursing aversion and agitation in breastfeeding mothers', *Iranian Journal of Nursing and Midwifery Research*, 22(6), pp. 449–454.

17 Ureño, T. L. *et al.* (2019) 'Dysphoric milk ejection reflex: A descriptive study', *Breastfeeding Medicine*, 14(9), pp. 666–673.

18 Heise, A. M. and Wiessinger, D. (2017) *Before The Letdown: Dysphoric Milk Ejection Reflex and the Breastfeeding Mother*. Edited by D. M. Watkinson. (Independently published)

19 Uvnas-Moberg, K. and Kendall-Tackett, K. (2018) 'The mystery of D-MER: What can hormonal research tell us about dysphoric milk-ejection reflex?', *Clinical Lactation*, 9(1), pp. 23–29.

20 Yate, Z. (2020) *When Breastfeeding Sucks: What You Need to Know about Nursing Aversion and Agitation*. London: Pinter & Martin.

21 Marasco, L. and West, D. (2019) *Making More Milk: The Breastfeeding Guide to Increasing Your Milk Production*. 2nd edn. New York: McGraw-Hill Education.

7 Does breastfeeding improve parental and infant mental health?

The birth of a baby is a challenging time for both parents' mental health as they face their new roles and responsibilities, as well as changing relationships. Some parents may have or can develop changes in their mental health during or after pregnancy. Others may develop symptoms after the birth, after several months, or at vulnerable points, such as returning to work. The onset of psychosis can be unexpected and sudden and will usually require hospital treatment. Parents who suffer from pre-existing mental health conditions can find their symptoms become more severe at this time. Commonly, community practitioners will find they are supporting many parents in their caseloads with postnatal anxiety and low mood. It is important, to recognise that perinatal depression can happen to men as well as women, but they are less likely to admit it or seek help from health visitors.

The experiences of babies in pregnancy, birth and early postnatal life can impact on their brain development, especially the emotional centres of their brains and subsequently their future mental health. Breastfeeding can lead to babies building close, loving relationships, bonding and secure attachment with their mothers, which can have a profound effect on their long-term mental health.

This chapter will explore some of the quantitative and qualitative evidence on how breastfeeding impacts mental health and how this can influence community practitioners' practice priorities.

Does breastfeeding help to protect mothers from perinatal depression?

Perinatal depression and anxiety are thought to affect 10–20%[1] of all mothers, so all community practitioners are likely to know women suffering from it at the moment. It ranges through a continuum of common worries about the health, safety and development of their babies, through to baby blues, irrational fears or obsessive, compulsive disorder, and to full psychosis. Health visitors, midwives and GPs are in positions, during their contacts in pregnancy and in the first postnatal months to pick up on worrying signs, by listening carefully to what the women are saying. There are both quantitative and qualitative research findings across the world that breastfeeding exclusively has a protective effect against perinatal mental health disorders. More recently, it has been recognised that it would be beneficial to integrate infant feeding support with mental health support, as one often impacts on the other.

What do quantitative studies tell us?

Several studies have been done that give us data from around the world on the impact of breastfeeding on mothers' mental health. These describe the impact on their mental

DOI: 10.4324/9781003139775-7

health of not being able to breastfeed, when they had intended to do so whilst pregnant.

Mothers' feeding intentions were evaluated in pregnancy by Borra[2] in a large study of 14,000 parents and their children in Bristol. Their mental health was measured using the Edinburgh Postnatal Depression Scale, at 8 weeks and 8, 21 and 32 months after their babies were born. This study found that the lowest rate of postpartum depression (PPD) was amongst women who had planned to breastfeed in pregnancy and had achieved their infant feeding goals. The highest risks of PPD were in those women who wanted to breastfeed but were unable to do so.

It was apparent that the impact of not being able to breastfeed when they intended to do so was profound and could lead to maternal depression. This paper also recommended the importance of providing expert breastfeeding support to all women who wish to breastfeed, together with compassionate support for mothers who intended to but found they were unable to do so.

Another study had similar findings – that when women have depressive symptoms in pregnancy, it can lead to high levels of these symptoms when they are not exclusively breastfeeding when their babies are 3 months old. Exclusive breastfeeding, however, at 3 months predicted continuation until 6 months and was associated with a reduced incidence of PPD. Early, especially antenatal identification of maternal depression and anxiety followed by offering additional support, promoted maternal well-being and prevented breastfeeding problems.[3]

Breastfeeding has also been shown to have a protective effect on other mental health disorders. A study carried out on 186,452 mothers in Australia showed that breastfeeding was associated with a decrease in hospital admissions for a variety of mental health conditions ranging from schizophrenia, bipolar affective disorder and mental illness associated with substance abuse in the first postpartum year.[4]

It is known that teenage parents and their infants are at high risk of poor physical and mental outcomes. A review article on young parents found that if maternal and paternal depression were recognised in pregnancy and additional support for breastfeeding given, then family well-being, attachment and infant mental health would be improved.[5]

This strong evidence shows that if we can identify anxiety and depression in pregnancy, we can tailor additional support to enable mothers to breastfeed exclusively and reduce the likelihood of severe mental health problems in the first 6 months after birth.

What additional insights do qualitative studies give us?

Qualitative studies of mothers' experiences give a more in-depth picture of their feelings but can only be done on smaller numbers. They use semi-structured interviews and observation to elicit the way mothers navigate their way through challenges they meet. They also help us to understand their lived experiences and give them time to express some of their deeper thoughts.

The perceptions of breastfeeding for women with perinatal depression and their embodied experiences were explored by studying ten women who had self-reported perinatal depression. They found some common themes which were that the women had feelings of inadequacy, but were deliberately persevering in a selfless way for the intimacy breastfeeding gave them with their babies. The researcher concluded that understanding the thoughts that women might have when depressed could help nurses and others working in mental health understand why optimum breastfeeding support would have a positive effect on mothers' psychological well-being.[6]

A systematic review of qualitative papers revealed similar themes expressed by the voices of women who became depressed, which are all particularly relevant for community practitioners and may already be familiar to you in your work with mothers suffering from postpartum mental health issues. It was found that many women with postnatal depression expressed the views that they had strong intentions to breastfeed and be 'good mothers', but if unable to do so, some perceived themselves as failures which triggered their mental health problems. The authors recommended that all parents receive practical and non-judgemental support from healthcare professionals, as well as from family and friends to support their mental health and infant feeding.[7]

Another informative qualitative, anthropological study was carried out on 17 mothers with babies in neonatal intensive care units. This study showed that this is a particularly difficult time for parents, because they are usually separated from their babies, who are very unwell or may not survive. It captured their stories of failure and guilt and suffering. Parents spoke of the trauma of being physically separated and unable to hold or breastfeed their babies, and their fractured relationships with them. They spoke of feeling marginalised from their infants' care and disempowered within the unit. The author suggested that NICUs are redesigned to prioritise mother–infant dyads' relationships and prioritise infants' and mothers' mental health.[8]

An online survey had similar findings that mothers who wished to breastfeed but find they are unable to meet their goals, may experience feelings of anxiety, guilt and anger which can lead to depression. The researcher in addition argued that breastfeeding advocates may be blamed for promoting breastfeeding with their focus on the baby, rather than the mother. She suggested that we all need to recognise and value every woman's breastfeeding wishes and not dismiss or invalidate their experiences by telling them that they do not matter.[9]

These quantitative and qualitative studies throw light on the experiences of women who become depressed after childbirth and how breastfeeding, especially exclusively, has a protective role on their mental health. Their infant feeding experiences will impact on their long-term relationships with their babies and partners. If we can identify risk factors in pregnancy, we could plan extra breastfeeding support for them before and immediately after their births. You could invite them to attend antenatal sessions and breastfeeding support groups when pregnant, where they could be introduced to specialists and peer supporters. I think we need to take a proactive approach in order to provide optimum support for their breastfeeding journey in order to protect their mental health.

Do we understand how breastfeeding protects mothers' mental health?

There is emerging evidence that depression is linked to inflammation in the body which could explain why psychosocial, behavioural and physical risk factors increase the risk of postnatal mental health problems. Cathy Kendall-Tackett argues that proinflammatory cytokines increase in women in the last trimester of pregnancy, and at this time there is a high risk of signs of depression.[10] She also says that the common experiences of new motherhood, such as sleep disturbance, postpartum pain, past or current psychological trauma can act as stressors and increase the risk of this inflammatory process. Breastfeeding has a protective effect on maternal mental health because it reduces stress and modulates this inflammatory response. It has a much larger role than just feeding babies because it helps to maintain and protect both physical and mental health. It increases maternal responsivity and connectivity resulting in the child developing secure attachment, reducing their stress levels as well. These responses to inflammation can lead mothers to experience a life of good health.

She argues, 'In short, breastfeeding can make the world a happier and healthier place', and that breastfeeding difficulties, such as nipple pain, can increase the risk of depression and must be addressed promptly. High quality breastfeeding support should be offered to all mothers, but particularly those where any risk factors for depression have been identified in pregnancy. This new paradigm can be used during antenatal and early postnatal contacts to identify women who might be at risk of developing this inflammatory response. They could then be prioritised for extra psychological support, in their transition to parenthood.

A mother's story of how breastfeeding helped her overcome her serious mental health problems

> Growing up I felt ashamed of my body. It betrayed me over and over again. I developed eating disorders and depression. I am skilled at self-harm, especially cutting. I have attempted suicide on a number of occasions. Planned it on more. I think we need to talk more about what breastfeeding is like for women who fear their bodies and ultimately how redemptive and healing breastfeeding can be.
>
> Predictably, when my breasts began developing, I was horrified. I was self-conscious and wished they would go away. At this time, I had no concept of breasts existing for the purpose of lactation. My developing breasts drew appraising looks from my father and I hated them for it.
>
> The eating disorders developed in my late teens. It started when I went to university. I was the first one in my family to attend a university and my mother disapproved. I was floundering and lost. Feeling the punishment of hunger felt good. Not eating more than I absolutely needed felt good. Vomiting after the weakness of succumbing to hunger felt good. I felt in control. Able to manipulate things other people couldn't. I felt somewhat of a superhero. This is when things become a little hazy due to severe weight loss. I do remember feeling pleased when my periods stopped. When I continued to lose weight, I would think pleasantly about how perfectly skinny my corpse would be. The less of me the better. Existing was painful. Being alive was painful. It was suffering. Cutting helped as a release, especially when I managed to get the slashes of the blade perfectly symmetrical to each other on my forearm or my thigh.
>
> So during my pregnancy I decided that I would give breastfeeding a go but if it didn't work out I wasn't going to do a number on myself. I wasn't going to be one of those women crying because of breastfeeding. I knew a bit about the value of breastmilk but knew no breastfeeding friends or family members. I knew I wasn't breastfed. It wasn't that big a deal. Right? I didn't do any breastfeeding education classes. It wasn't something that women like me did. In late pregnancy I found colostrum leaking from my breasts. I was actually repulsed. I hated that I had no control over my breasts. I felt betrayed. I told no one and pretended that I hadn't seen anything. Must. Maintain. Control.
>
> So my son was born. Not the birth I planned. I thought he was kind of a bit cute but there was no rush of love. In Recovery I offered him my breast and he latched. He liked being at the breast. The first night in hospital I spent the entire night with him in bed with me and he was latched on. I had no idea of normal baby behaviour or anything like building a supply. I just thought he was a weirdo but went with it. When a midwife

popped her head round the door in the middle of the night I thought she would tell me off for having the baby in bed with me but she just smiled warmly and left. I felt safe. She didn't even say anything. She just smiled at me and it was a massive comfort.

The next day I began to doubt my milk supply and a different midwife suggested offering a bottle of formula. So I did. Or rather I tried. My one-day-old son was extremely insistent that he did not want to drink from a bottle. I couldn't believe it. How many new-born babies turn their nose up at a bottle? How could he be so certain that he wanted to breastfeed? It seems I had been blessed with the smartest baby in the world. I had no choice. I had to breastfeed. And I did. I was uncertain about it. There were many doubts. But I did it. When my nipples were sore my mother bought me nipple cream and never once suggested formula. I remain perplexed by how out of character this really was. But pleased. I developed a Mummy friendship with an amazing woman. She was breastfeeding her daughter and we shared a similar bitter sense of humour. She kept me going. She tells me now that I kept her going.

It wasn't all rosy. Unsurprisingly there was some post natal depression, but my mother is Irish and I have inherited the luck of the Irish. I had an amazing health visitor and she supported me with some CBT: the depression was mild and transient. She encouraged me to train as a peer supporter.

I am still incredulous that I was able to provide my beautiful son with the sole source of his nutrition. For 6 months. And I continued to breastfeed him until he was 19 months old. My body did that. My breasts did that. It's incredible. It's somewhat unbelievable at times but it's incredible. I can't fathom why we don't talk about anything other than the wonder of breasts. I feel sorry for the people who will never get to transfer this life sustaining fluid to someone they love. I feel blessed and privileged and extremely lucky. And grateful. Being able to breastfeed was the most influential factor on how I felt about my body. It was more effective than years of counselling and medications. I know it's not going to be that simple for everyone, but I strongly believe that we need to talk more about this. How do we reach those women who doubt their bodies and who don't have babies who refuse bottles of formula? How often do we talk to women about how they felt about their body growing up? Isn't that the beginning of the process that will determine a woman's chances of breastfeeding success?

Can breastfeeding help protect father's mental health too?

Although fathers cannot breastfeed, they can have skin-to-skin contact with their babies which brings feelings of closeness and bonding with the high oxytocin levels that they and their babies make, which can lead to strong feelings of well-being. Fathers and partners can connect with babies through caring, bathing, carrying, speaking, singing, reading and settling them. Babies are familiar with their voices already, having heard them throughout pregnancy, and often feel very secure when they are held close to their bodies, or will calm down when fussy and relax. This is such an important role as most babies have unsettled times during the day or night!

Community practitioners can prepare parents for those unsettled times which may begin soon after birth, but sometimes become worse at 2–3 weeks. Commonly babies want to breastfeed frequently on the second night, which can be challenging for tired mothers, but they can be reassured that this will help to establish their milk supply. Then, subsequently, they have appetite spurts at 3 weeks and 6 weeks when they want to feed more often for a few days. Fathers' or partners' understanding of these means they will be able to offer mothers the reassurance that their milk is providing everything their babies need, so long as they are feeding effectively. Their influence is profound and will make all the difference to breastfeeding continuing or not.

What do we know about fathers' mental health in their transition to parenthood?

Research on new fathers shows that 5–18% of them will suffer from perinatal depression especially those who are vulnerable to depression and anxiety beforehand. Poor mental health of fathers can impact on partners, children and society and is a major public health issue that does not receive the attention it deserves. The effects can be long term and impact on infant and child development, and there is evidence that severe depression can lead to psychiatric, behavioural and conduct disorders in children at 7 years.[11]

A systematic review of qualitative papers on fathers around the world[12] found insights into what men experience in their transition to parenthood. The main themes centred around new fatherhood identity, the competing challenges of new fatherhood, their negative feelings and fears, stress they encountered and problems coping with it, particularly the lack of support they found. The three main factors affecting men's mental health were whether they were able to find their new fatherhood identity, the competing challenges they met and whether they were able to overcome their negative fears and feelings.

Expectant and new fathers experienced a range of fears around not knowing what to expect in labour and birth and looking after a new baby and how they would be able to balance the competing demands of work and supporting the physical and emotional needs of their new family. They also felt unprepared for the changes in their relationships with their partners while they were focussing on those of their babies and some resorted to denial and escape activities such as smoking or working longer hours.

Many men in the UK experienced a lack of support from health visitors, which they saw as a service given by women for women and the lack of father-friendly resources available. Many men felt positively about their new identity as they found they were fulfilling their role as men and recognised their new roles and responsibilities, but some worried about getting it right.

This study also found that many fathers reported that breastfeeding was harder than they anticipated and felt unprepared, helpless and useless, when they could not help. They often found that healthcare professionals had not been honest and they were not told antenatally that breastfeeding could be very painful if their babies had not been latched on well. Some felt unprepared about the frequency of feeds, with one running into the next with no respite. These findings suggest that giving positive support to fathers, would increase their knowledge, attitudes to breastfeeding and ability to provide practical and emotional support to their partners.

There is an opportunity here for antenatal and postnatal services to become more targeted at both parents, so fathers feel involved in preparation for breastfeeding, knowledgeable about the way babies achieve good milk transfer and how to support their partners in the early days and months of their children's lives.

Discussions could be focussed on how they can adjust emotionally to their new role and bond with their new babies, as well as information about practical help and support they can give their partners. You could emphasise their important role in comforting and settling their babies when they are distressed, helping to assess effective milk transfer, by observing feeds and monitoring nappy outputs.

They can be given information on additional sources of support if needed, from the local infant feeding teams, support from breastfeeding charities, and evidence-based apps such as Baby Buddy, which now has targeted information for fathers. They can also contact the National Breastfeeding Helpline and talk to breastfeeding counsellors directly if their partners are reluctant to do so.

Has the COVID-19 pandemic had an impact on parents' mental health?

The recent Royal Foundation Report (2020)[13] demonstrated that the COVID-19 pandemic has exacerbated the mental health crisis in the UK. It was found that 38–63% of parents told them that their loneliness had increased after the first lockdown. It made a recommendation that parents and carers of small children needed more support and advice to ensure their optimal mental health.

A recent online survey of 1,219 women after the first national lockdown in 2020 found that 41.8% thought that their breastfeeding had been protected because they had more time at home with their partners and new baby and were not under pressure to have visitors. However, 27% struggled to get enough support from professionals and families and stopped breastfeeding before they were ready. These women were more likely to come from BAME groups, live in challenging circumstances and have lower educational achievements. They may be more likely to suffer from guilt, loss and depression as they were unable to breastfeed for as long as they wished.[14]

This pandemic has shown that BAME groups have been disproportionately seriously affected by this novel virus and death rates have been higher. The EMBRACE report showed that Black African women are five times more likely to die in childbirth and Asian women three times more likely than white women. Inequalities in mental health are profound, affecting access, experience and outcomes. NHS England has developed a strategy to reduce mental health inequalities:

> Tackling inequalities, especially racism, is vital, emotive and challenging. It requires leaders, organisations and individuals to understand their own biases, beliefs and behaviours. It requires every component of the systems we operate within to acknowledge the stark reality of inequality. We will only tackle inequalities by understanding people's experience of them and acting to change.[15]

It also recommends suitable therapies for individuals from BAME groups who generally have poorer recovery rates from talking therapies, such as counselling, than white-British ones.

It is important to recognise different racial and socio-economic groups have different likelihoods of developing mental health problems which may be influenced by multiple personal, social and environmental factors. As an example, people who have adverse childhood experiences are more likely than others to develop mental health problems. Parents with existing mental health problems are likely to need extra support with breastfeeding their babies.

The 'Babies in Lockdown' report also came from an online survey of 5,474 parents and showed how families at risk of poorer outcomes suffered the most during the first lockdown. This is likely to widen the deep inequalities which already exist in early life experiences and life chances; 60% were concerned about their own and their children's mental health, as they struggled with the challenges of feeding and caring for their new babies, causing an increase in their anxiety levels. Only 10% were able to have face-to-face support from their health visitors and many felt 'abandoned' or that they were 'falling through the cracks'. Although 55% were breastfeeding, over half of them were giving formula, although they had not intended to do so. The recommendations to Government from this report were to increase support to protect the mental health of parents and their children, especially in these vulnerable groups with a significant and sustained investment in services from conception to aged two.[16]

The NHS Long Term Plan ambitions for mental health sets the expectation that all systems need to reduce mental health inequalities by 2023/24.[17] Community practitioners have a key role in this, to listen to and support parents in the perinatal period, enabling them to achieve their infant feeding goals and protect their mental health and that of their babies.

It is likely that the pandemic will have long-term effects on parents' and their children's mental health, leading to growing inequalities in health, unless the government gives additional resources to target them. As community practitioners, often working with large caseloads, we can do our best to ensure that all new families receive optimum support with breastfeeding, which will enable them to benefit from the protective, restorative effect it can have on their mental health.

What do we know about how infants' mental health develops?

In the last 20 years we have learned a great deal about how babies' brains are affected by their experiences in utero and after birth, through neuropsychology, epigenetics, psycho- history and anthropology. The evidence base is growing rapidly, but I will attempt to summarise the main themes from four academics who have looked at the impact of skin-to-skin, breastfeeding and children's experiences on their mental health. They come from medical, psychological and sociological backgrounds and looked at how the child's future mental health is affected during pregnancy and by their early experiences after birth and into childhood and beyond.

Nils Bergman was one of the first clinicians to talk about the vital importance of 'nil separation' between mothers and babies after birth, in his work on 'kangaroo mother care' for pre-term babies.[18] Here he argues that babies' experiences of pregnancy, birth and breastfeeding 'wire and fire' neural circuits in their brains, with their sleep being important in this process, especially the long sleep most have after the birth. The mother's body provides the environment for new-born infants, especially in skin contact, with the smell of her areolar glands eliciting her baby's emotional and bonding behaviour. This influences high oxytocin levels and changes in the amygdala, an emotional centre in the brain, leading to epigenetic changes and the way the baby's DNA is expressed in developing social behaviour. He claims that maternal support in the early days and weeks after childbirth will predict larger hippocampal volumes in the child at school age. This critical opportunity in early life, when a child's brain is primed to receive sensory input, will lead to more advanced neural systems developing. He also argues that a child can suffer from toxic stress when separated from his mother, which can lead to a rise in cortisol and a reduction in oxytocin levels. If this is sustained over time and not buffered by a supportive relationship, it can lead to stress-related physical and mental illness.

Bergman's vision is:

A world where every baby at birth stays in skin-to-skin contact with mother, and can begin breastfeeding and bonding naturally, and go on to establish a secure attachment relationship for a better society.

His film on 'Grow your Baby's Brain'[19] describes how breastfeeding and skin-to-skin contact with mother is the first stimulus for the amygdala-prefrontal tract, which he claims is the first pathway for a healthy right brain and emotional development, leading to secure attachment and subsequent positive mental health outcomes.

Robin Grille, an Australian psychotherapist, has looked at children's mental health through neuropsychology, epigenetics, psychohistory and anthropology and how cultures have lost the capacity for healthy attachment. He also talks about the importance of oxytocin as a 'fertiliser' of the brain and how it gives both the mother and her child a profound sense of well-being, closeness and bliss, which is shared as they build responsive attachment.

He claims that the breastfeeding mother's brain actually gains weight due to her high oxytocin levels as she connects with her child, and builds empathy and responsive attachment resulting in increased emotional intelligence. He says that parents are the 'empathy farmers' of the next generation. If they can avoid the build-up of cortisol, a neuro toxin, through harsh, punitive parenting, they can prevent damage to the prefrontal region of the child's brain leading to less violent and aggressive behaviour in later childhood and adult life. He argues in his book *Parenting for a Peaceful World* that he sees a world full of societies of empathy which are harmonious and peaceful about which he spoke in his lecture to the Baby Friendly Conference in 2015.[20]

Karleen Gribble who is an Australian professor of nursing has similarly suggested that close skin-to-skin contact between mothers and their infants leads them both to experience high levels of the hormone oxytocin, which in turn reduces the stress hormone cortisol that can last for up to two days. Prolactin and cholecystokinin are also hormones that mothers release as the babies suckle on their breasts, helping them to relax, as well as reducing any pain they may be experiencing. Through these physiological and psychological processes mothers and babies develop close attachment. Gribble says that:

> Children who have experienced consistent, responsive, care-giving, develop a positive internal working model of relationships and a high level of personal value, both of which are building blocks for success in future relationships.[21]

Another Australian study looked at the long-term effects of breastfeeding on a child's and adolescent's mental health through a longitudinal study of 2,900 women and their children up to 14 years, which showed that children who were breastfed for less than 6 months had poorer mental health outcomes throughout childhood and adolescence.[22]

It has also been demonstrated in a study in the USA of depressed mothers' interactions with their babies, that breastfeeding increased the number of times they touched each other, boosted babies' mood and changed their brain function.[23]

What are the conclusions we can draw from this research?

Women's mental health is improved if they receive consistent, informed, accessible support, enabling them to breastfeed and achieve their infant feeding goals. Fathers or partners also need support while they adjust to parenthood and go through the liminal time after birth, when they leave their previous life behind and may need time to talk about their feelings, especially as their relationship as a couple changes. This support needs to begin in pregnancy with a discussion about breastfeeding, including realistic expectations of new-born babies' behaviour, their needs for skin-to-skin closeness and building close relationships with them. After birth, active listening to their stories will help them clarify their experiences and identify any breastfeeding or mental health challenges, referring them to specialist services when appropriate. We need to be aware that families from BAME communities may find it more difficult to access services or may not want to admit to symptoms of depression.

When breastfeeding does not work or mothers decide to change to bottle feeding, they may experience a lowering of mood with the reduction in oxytocin. It could be helpful to suggest they have more skin-to-skin contact, keep their babies close and give them lots of cuddles to give this hormone a boost, which may help to reduce their feelings of loss and grief and is likely to help their mental health and their relationship with their babies.

The evidence above has shown that babies' brains are sensitive to parents' emotions in utero and after birth; while building close, loving relationships, oxytocin levels rise, which 'fertilise' their neurons by 'wiring' and 'firing' them to develop trust, empathy and positive psychological attachment. As Grille and Bergman suggest, parents have a vital role in developing their babies' brains. Mothers' mental health improves with breastfeeding through the benefits of the hormone prolactin and cholecystokinin, which are thought to increase mothering behaviours and close attachment. If children do not receive this nurturing environment to build close, loving relationships with their parents, this could have a negative impact on their physical and mental development and lead to problems in later life.

Through this close association between positive breastfeeding experiences and good mental health, there could be an argument to integrate the two support strategies, and perhaps in the future to think about training women and men to become breastfeeding/perinatal peer supporters.

What are the implications of this research for community practitioners?

As I have shown above, there is now a very strong evidence base on the links between exclusive breastfeeding and the protection it can give to parents' perinatal mental health. It demonstrates that prioritising optimum support for parents with breastfeeding is crucial for their present and future mental health. When community practitioners can introduce new mothers and fathers to the local infant feeding support networks, ideally in pregnancy, it will enable them to find information, meet other mothers and peers, and enable them to access support with breastfeeding, leading to positive mental health outcomes for the whole family.

Notes

1 Kendall-Tackett, K. (2007) 'A new paradigm for depression in new mothers: The central role of inflammation and how breastfeeding and anti-inflammatory treatments protect maternal mental health', *International Breastfeeding Journal*, 2, p. 6.
2 Borra, C., Iacovou, M. and Sevilla, A. (2015) 'New evidence on breastfeeding and post-partum depression: The importance of understanding women's intentions', *Maternal and Child Health Journal*, 19(4), pp. 897–907.
3 Coo, S. *et al.* (2020) 'The role of perinatal anxiety and depression in breastfeeding practices', *Breastfeeding Medicine: The Official Journal of the Academy of Breastfeeding Medicine*, 15 (8), pp. 495–500.

4 Xu, F. *et al.* (2014) 'Does infant feeding method impact on maternal mental health?', *Breastfeeding Medicine: The Official Journal of the Academy of Breastfeeding Medicine*, 9(4), pp. 215–221.

5 McPeak, K. E. *et al.* (2015) 'Important determinants of newborn health: Postpartum depression, teen parenting, and breast-feeding', *Current Opinion in Pediatrics*, 27(1), pp. 138–144.

6 Pratt, B. A. *et al.* (2020) 'Perceptions of breastfeeding for women with perinatal depression: A descriptive phenomenological study', *Issues in Mental Health Nursing*, 41(7), pp. 637–644.

7 Tanganhito, D. D. S., Bick, D. and Chang, Y.-S. (2020) 'Breastfeeding experiences and perspectives among women with postnatal depression: A qualitative evidence synthesis', *Women and Birth*, 33(3), pp. 231–239.

8 Palmquist, A. E. L., Holdren, S. M. and Fair, C. D. (2020) '"It was all taken away": Lactation, embodiment, and resistance among mothers caring for their very-low-birth-weight infants in the neonatal intensive care unit', *Social Science & Medicine*, 244, p. 112648.

9 Brown, A. (2018) 'What do women lose if they are prevented from meeting their breastfeeding goals?', *Clinical Lactation*, 9(4), pp. 200–207.

10 Kendall-Tackett, K. (2007) 'A new paradigm for depression in new mothers: The central role of inflammation and how breastfeeding and anti-inflammatory treatments protect maternal mental health', *International Breastfeeding Journal*, 2, p. 6.

11 Ramchandani, P. G. *et al.* (2013) 'Do early father–infant interactions predict the onset of externalising behaviours in young children? Findings from a longitudinal cohort study', *Journal of Child Psychology and Psychiatry*, 54(1), pp. 56–64.

12 Baldwin, S. *et al.* (2018) 'Mental health and wellbeing during the transition to fatherhood: A systematic review of first time fathers' experiences', *JBI Evidence Synthesis*, 16(11), pp. 2118–2191.

13 Royal Foundation (2020) *The Duchess of Cambridge and The Royal Foundation Release the #5BigInsights in The Biggest Ever Study on the Early Years*. Available at: https://royalfoundation.com/the-duchess-of-cambridge-unveils-five-big-insights-research-early-years/

14 Brown, A. and Shenker, N. (2021) 'Experiences of breastfeeding during COVID-19: Lessons for future practical and emotional support', *Maternal & Child Nutrition*, 17(1), p. e13088.

15 NHS England (2020) *Advancing Mental Health Equalities Strategy*. Available at: www.england.nhs.uk/publication/advancing-mental-health-equalities-strategy/

16 Babies in Lockdown (2020) *Babies in Lockdown*. Available at: https://babiesinlockdown.info/

17 NHS England (2019) *Adult Mental Health Services: Long Term Plan*. Available at: www.longtermplan.nhs.uk/online-version/chapter-3-further-progress-on-care-quality-and-outcomes/better-care-for-major-health-conditions/adult-mental-health-services/

18 Bergman, N. J. (2004) 'Kangaroo Mother Care: The importance of skin-to-skin contact'. *British Medical Journal*, 329, p. 1179. Available at: www.bmj.com/rapid-response/2011/10/30/kangaroo-mother-care-importance-skin-skin-contact

19 See www.geddesproduction.com/product/grow-your-babys-brain/

20 Grille, R. (2015) 'Neuro-social evolution'. *Baby Friendly Initiative*. Available at: www.unicef.org.uk/babyfriendly/baby-friendly-resources/relationship-building-resources/robin-grille-neuro-social-evolution-video/

21 Gribble, K. D. (2006) 'Mental health, attachment and breastfeeding: Implications for adopted children and their mothers', *International Breastfeeding Journal*, 1, p. 5.

22 Oddy, W. H. *et al.* (2010) 'The long-term effects of breastfeeding on child and adolescent mental health: A pregnancy cohort study followed for 14 years', *The Journal of Pediatrics*, 156(4), pp. 568–574.

23 Schmidt, C. E. (2021) 'Depressed moms who breastfeed boost babies' mood, neuroprotection and mutual touch'. *ScienceDaily*. Available at: www.sciencedaily.com/releases/2021/02/210210091209.htm

8 Health visitors just weigh babies!

Health visitors' baby clinics are sometimes seen by parents as places where they can just weigh their babies, but we all know they are so much more than that. They can be important contact times, when there can be discussions about children's growth, development, skin rashes, introducing solid foods, potty training, behaviour problems in toddlers etc. Parents may also talk of any problems they may have with their own mental health, or their relationships with their partners or children, which may require follow-up home visits. The list of issues is endless, but all part of the holistic supportive care health visitors offer to parents.

In this chapter, I will suggest ways of assessing breastfeeding without relying on weighing babies. These should be shared with parents, so they can identify any problems early and gradually trust the process and build their own self-reliance.

Frequent weighing of breastfed infants can be problematic, because it can undermine parents' confidence, especially if they compare their babies with others who may also be breastfed or formula fed. The other consideration is that babies tend to grow in spurts, not usually in a uniform way, and frequent feeding at these times may be interpreted by mothers and health visitors that their milk supplies are inadequate, rather than just the way babies are responding to their need for more calories for growth.

Do most women make enough breastmilk for their babies?

In our culture today, breastfeeding may be seen by parents and professionals as unreliable because, as I have discussed earlier, over the past three generations of formula feeding we have become used to measuring the volumes of milk babies are consuming. We have no way of telling how much a baby is taking from the breast! We do know that the large majority of mothers make plenty of milk for their babies, if they are given adequate support and accurate information on attaching their babies correctly onto their breasts. Their milk supplies are stimulated by frequent, effective feeding and keeping their babies close to stimulate their hormone responses.

In many countries in the world where breastfeeding is the normal way, babies are fed and have free access to the breast 24 hours a day; no one worries about the volumes of milk they are consuming. A mother who had exclusively breastfed her first two babies for over 2 years in Brazil and had just given birth to her third baby in London told me:

> I think in the UK you only worry about the baby's weight, not how he is fed! My midwife has just told me that because my 10-day-old baby is not back to his birth weight that I need to give him formula top ups. I told her that I want to breastfeed, so I do not want to give him artificial milk.

DOI: 10.4324/9781003139775-8

The arrival of a new baby in the UK is often announced with his or her gender and weight! Everyone wants to know if the baby is healthy and they judge this by his or her weight. A child's subsequent weight gain has been given social meaning as an indicator of good parenting. In the past, parents and families have assumed that babies who gain weight quickly are healthy, but now there are concerns that rapid growth in early childhood may predispose to childhood and lifelong obesity and ill health as an adult.

In this chapter, I will look at evidence in the NICE guideline on faltering growth and consider the expected 'normal' growth parameters in the time after birth and the first year of life and discuss how breastfeeding should be protected as the physiological norm. I will then suggest ways of assessing breastfeeds by observing babies' positioning and attachment on the breasts to ensure they are obtaining effective milk transfer.

How can we tell how much a baby is taking from the breast?

We need to look at the *baby's behaviour* on the breast and after feeds, as well as other *signs of milk transfer*. In Chapter 5, I looked at the way a baby is positioned and attached to the breast to ensure a good flow of milk during a feed, if her mouth is not taking a wide, deep mouthful of areola, which is in an asymmetrical latch, she will be unable to draw adequate milk from the breast. Parents can assess how their babies are feeding by seeing the long, drawing sucks, with their jaws, with bouts interspersed with pauses and can usually hear their babies swallowing! Babies then come off the breast spontaneously by releasing the suction and moving their heads away or falling asleep and releasing the breast. If they have taken enough milk to fill their tummies, they will look full and often 'milk drunk'. Many babies will want to take the second breast just to finish. Parents can be reassured by observing the urine and stools output as well (see Figure 5.15).

This scenario where babies are not adequately latched, are unsettled and not gaining weight, is sadly all too common, especially in the early weeks, but the reason for this is usually poor positioning and attachment on the breasts. Once you know what to look for it will become second nature for you so you will be able to give parents the support and information they need to gain confidence.

As I discussed in Chapter 5, if babies are not positioned with their noses level with the nipples, they cannot take a large enough mouthful of breast tissue to transfer the milk from the breast to the back of their mouths effectively (see Figure 5.13).

You could observe the way the mother holds her baby and positions her baby for breastfeeding. It may be that her nipple is aimed to the centre of the baby's mouth, so you could suggest that she moves the baby across her body away from the breast she is using, so the head is tilted back (not held) with her nose level with the nipple.

Make sure the baby is held very close and facing her body. Baby's body needs to be in a straight line and usually held below the breast, often at an angle of 45 degrees. The mother can move her quickly to the breast with a wide mouth and her chin leading. Once she has taken a large mouthful of breast tissue and her chin is indenting the breast, she will take the nipple and lower areola into her mouth, with the mother's nipple being drawn along the roof of her mouth to the junction of the soft palate. She will then make deep jaw movements, with pauses and swallowing can usually be heard (see Figure 5.12 a–h).

The NICE Faltering Growth guideline committee (2017) considered 'normal' weight loss in the early weeks after birth and advised on the expected time for this to be regained by reviewing the literature systematically; they considered the cost effectiveness and included the following:

- The timing of maximal weight loss reported by six studies (119,676 infants) was 2–3 days after birth, regardless of feeding type.
- There was little difference in the maximum weight loss of exclusively breastfed and formula fed babies.
- It was found that babies delivered by caesarean section were likely to lose more weight in their first week, possibly because their mothers received intravenous fluids before delivery, so their birthweight was artificially high and this excess weight was lost in the first 3 days of life.
- Most babies stop losing weight at 3–4 days after birth.
- The threshold for 'normal' weight loss in the first week is 10% of birthweight.
- Most babies have regained their birthweight by 3 weeks.[1]

Excessive weight loss in the first week of life naturally causes parental anxiety and can result in supplementation of breastfeeds with formula milk. There are a few medical reasons why this may be indicated, such as if the baby is dehydrated or severely jaundiced or the mother cannot express sufficient milk. Mothers' expressed milk is always the best option when possible, because it will be better absorbed by the baby and the expressing will stimulate her milk production. In some hospitals, donor milk may be available if the mother is unable to express adequate volumes of her own milk. If babies' stomachs are stretched by larger volumes of formula given by bottle, they will be less satisfied by smaller volumes of colostrum/transitional milk, which may lead to less parental confidence in breastfeeding.

Most mothers do make plenty of breastmilk and, providing babies are feeding effectively through optimum positioning and attachment, they will obtain good milk transfer.

If you have any concerns about faltering growth, the NICE guidelines should be followed. These points should also be considered:

- ineffective suckling in breastfed infants
- ineffective bottle feeding
- feeding patterns or routines being used
- the feeding environment
- parent/carer–infant interactions
- how parents or carers respond to the infant's feeding cues
- physical disorders that affect feeding
- feeding aversion.

The NICE guidance for babies who have lost over 10%

- A full assessment of baby's general health and breastfeeding technique should be carried out by a fully trained person (at least to UNICEF Baby Friendly standards) to optimise adequate milk transfer.
- A care plan should be started but if there is no improvement in the baby's weight after these adjustments, additional expressed breastmilk should be given after breastfeeds, or formula milk if the mother finds it difficult to express.

- If a baby has lost just over 10% but otherwise assessed to be healthy, weight should be re-measured at 3 weeks.
- Exclusively breastfed infants should regain their birthweight by the time they are 3 weeks.

Many healthcare professionals are still not following these guidelines fully, expecting babies to regain their birthweight by 2 weeks, and recommend supplementary formula feeds before 3 weeks. This practice often leads to mothers making smaller volumes of breastmilk, because their babies are feeding less on their breasts, and not stimulating their supplies. This results in mothers having lower prolactin (the milk-making hormone) levels and finding they have inadequate milk supplies to satisfy their babies.

In the early days, if babies are not transferring adequate breastmilk when breastfeeding directly, it is very important that mothers express their milk frequently with a double, hospital grade breast pump, at least every three hours in the day and night, to build up and maintain their milk supplies. These breast pumps can be hired from the main manufacturers, which is a cheaper option.

Breastfeeding should always be protected when possible and mothers given optimum support to do so, when this is their chosen method of feeding, by referring to local support networks. Referrals to paediatric services should be made if there is any evidence of illness, marked weight loss or a failure to respond to feeding support – see NICE's guideline on postnatal care up to 8 weeks after birth.[2]

The thresholds for concern in milk fed babies under 6 months are:

- a fall across 1 or more weight centile spaces, if birthweight was below the 9th centile
- a fall across 2 or more weight centile spaces, if birthweight was between the 9th and 91st centiles
- a fall across 3 or more weight centile spaces, if birthweight was above the 91st centile
- when current weight is below the 2nd centile for age, whatever the birthweight.

(NB: One centile space being the space between adjacent centile lines.)

If you have concerns about faltering growth, you will need to monitor the weight carefully, but be aware that weighing children more frequently than is needed may add to parental anxiety (for example, minor short-term changes in weight may cause unnecessary concern). Remember that mothers usually make plenty of breastmilk for their babies and it is important to look at the positioning and attachment to ensure that babies are getting good milk transfer. If you have concerns that they are not after you have done a full feeding assessment, then you could support the mother to hand-express or pump her milk to supplement the feeds. This will stimulate her supply and ensure she can continue to breastfeed in the future, as well as give the baby some extra nutrition until she can latch and transfer milk more effectively.[3]

How can we assess breastfeeding without weighing the baby?

After the COVID-19 pandemic, the routine weighing of babies and young children is likely to become less frequent, as it is already in many European countries. If your assessment of breastfeeding positioning, attachment and milk transfer was satisfactory and parents are monitoring babies' behaviour, urine and stools output in the first 3 weeks, it is likely that babies are receiving plenty of milk. If you have assessed this to be happening, then monthly weights could be offered as a maximum, unless faltering growth has been identified.

What do babies' nappies tell us in the first week?

Most babies lose weight in the first 3 days after birth and are usually not weighed again until they are 5 days old. Parents can judge on a daily basis how well their babies are breastfeeding by observing their urine and stools output. It is important to share this information with parents in the antenatal period, as it helps them gain confidence as they start their breastfeeding journeys in the first week after the births of their babies.

Later on, usually after 8–10 weeks, breastfed babies may not pass stools every day, sometimes not for a week or even longer which is not constipation, but a normal physiological process, where they are just absorbing more of the breastmilk and there is little wastage. Parents do not need to worry about the baby being constipated because when they do pass stools they are likely to be soft and fairly runny as usual.

Over the following days, weeks and months babies tend to gain weight following their own centile lines, sometimes deviating slightly above or below, but should not fall more than two lines. Growth is determined by genetic factors and not just feeding, so the parents' average size should be taken into account.

Why supplementing with formula is often unhelpful when establishing breastfeeding

Mothers may be told in hospital by doctors or midwives that they are not making enough milk for their babies and are advised to supplement breastfeeds with formula milk. This may be justified in situations where babies are not latching on their mothers' breasts effectively and they struggle to express sufficient colostrum or milk. If faltering growth has been identified, then supplementation with expressed milk or formula, after breastfeeds, will be advised.

Healthy, new-born babies are often sleepy after birth, as I discussed in the last chapter, especially if their mothers have received drugs in labour. If this is the case, then mothers may ask for support to make sure they stimulate their breastmilk supplies by hand-expressing as soon and frequently as possible. Colostrum is best expressed by hand because it is thick and sticky and present in small volumes for the first two days after birth, but is very important for babies' immature gut, and gives them high protein feeds, full of antibodies, like a first immunisation protecting them from infection.

If babies continue to have problems latching on the breasts, then breast pumps can be used once mothers are hand-expressing more than 10ml at each expression, which is usually after two days. Frequent expressing either by hand or pump, that is at least 8–10 times in 24 hours, will help to establish mothers' milk supplies. They can continue with skin-to-skin to encourage babies' instinctive behaviour to attach to their breasts. Once they find the volume of expressed breastmilk is increasing, mothers begin to gain confidence that they are making plenty of breastmilk for their babies. They can be reassured that by establishing their milk supplies early, their babies will eventually latch and breastfeed directly. This is a stressful time for new parents during which it is important that they receive consistent, empathic support from midwives and their assistants, and peer supporters.

When babies are latching on the breasts, but appear hungry after feeds, or lose excessive weight, the likelihood is that they are *not positioning or attaching well* on their mothers' breasts, not that mothers are not making enough milk. You can share the information above and in Chapter 5, on effective positioning and attachment of their babies.

Can women who are supplementing change to breastfeeding exclusively?

How can women get out of this top up trap? They can stimulate their milk supplies to breastfeed exclusively, which is easier to do in the first few weeks. It is common for women to come home from hospital with their new babies breastfeeding and supplementing some or all feeds with formula milk and they may feel disappointment because they had intended to breastfeed exclusively. Unless the hospital is Baby Friendly accredited, expressed colostrum or breastmilk may not have been suggested and the mother may not have had enough support when attempting to latch her baby on her breasts.

This scenario is all too common, which is very unfortunate because it results in the breasts not being stimulated enough by the baby, as formula milk will fill her tummy and take time to digest, so she will not feed so well at the next breastfeed, and her mother's breastmilk production will reduce (Figure 8.1). If supplementing, she will need to express as well; in order to get out of this trap you can support the mother and build her confidence by trying the following:

- Observe her positioning and attaching her baby (as described in Chapter 5) and suggest adjustments if required.
- Encourage as much skin-to-skin contact as possible.
- Listen to her feelings, empathise with her situation and enable her to build her confidence in her ability to breastfeed exclusively.
- Support her to express her milk by hand or pump (or a mixture of the two), for short frequent periods, preferably after breastfeeds to stimulate her supply.
- Replace the formula supplements with breastmilk.
- Gradually stop supplements and put baby to her breasts frequently (often mothers find the early morning top ups can be stopped first and milk production is highest at night and in the early morning).
- Encourage her to monitor her baby's urine and stool output and weight if she has lost excessive amounts.
- Signpost her to mothers' support groups or peer support, face-to-face, or Facebook groups online.
- Give her information on the National Breastfeeding Helpline and very helpful apps such Baby Buddy.

Two very different mothers' stories about how they stopped supplements

This first story is when her baby had low blood sugar measurements:

> As my son weighed over 11lb at birth his blood sugar was constantly tested post-delivery. After having successfully given him his first feed at the breast, I was advised to provide him with formula as he had a low blood sugar level. As soon as

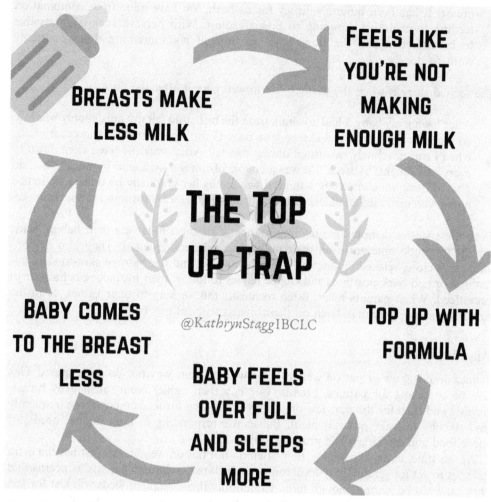

Figure 8.1 The top up trap
Source: Courtesy of Kathryn Stagg IBCLC.

he was introduced to the bottle he developed more or less instant nipple confusion and thereafter refused the breast altogether. I was in complete despair as I really wanted to breastfeed. For two and a half months I exclusively pumped my breastmilk for him, weaning him off of any formula altogether. Exclusively pumping was thoroughly exhausting but I was committed to providing him with breastmilk for better nutrition and immunity. I would wake up every two or three hours even when my son was asleep to pump, in order to provide him with sufficient milk. At first I could barely express 20ml or 30ml and I thought I would never be able to breastfeed him again. Constantly pumping a minimum of 8 to 10 times a day helped me to increase my supply such that I was able to pump around 300ml in the morning from both breasts. One day, when I took my son into the bath with me, he latched, on his own terms by himself. I have now managed to bring him back to the breast entirely. Ironically, he now sometimes refuses the bottle for the breast! It has been quite a journey for us both. We have gone from combination feeding to exclusive pumping to breastfeeding. With perseverance it is possible to breastfeed again. So, don't give up hope if it's something that you really want to do.

The second story is when the mother was unwell herself after the birth:

After having my baby, I had anaemia from the birth and felt my milk supply was low. At night for the first two weeks we gave baby G top ups of formula and occasionally when I was absolutely exhausted during the day. After week 3/4 these went down to every other night, by week 5 it was a couple of times a week and by week 7 we had phased them out completely. I think it was seeing her gradually become more settled along with increased confidence in breastfeeding that meant we could phase them out.

Both these stories demonstrate the importance of mothers following their babies' leads and at the same time ensuring their milk supplies are stimulated. They also demonstrate that close, relaxed contact between the mother and her baby in skin-to-skin, co-bathing or laid-back positions will enable babies to follow their instinctive behaviour to breastfeed. When parents relax, listen to music, talk or sing to their babies, as in the first story above, they may latch on their breasts without any help.

Appetite spurts

Babies do not grow or put on weight or grow in a linear way but do so in spurts! This can be confusing for parents, because one day their babies seem satisfied by breast-feeding and then for the next few days, they are asking for feeds much more frequently and starting to wake more at night. Babies are responding to their bodies' needs for more food and calories, while growing longer.

At this time, in my experience, they often do not put on weight, but just use the extra calories to get longer and may look thinner, which may reinforce parents' concerns that they may not be getting enough milk. Commonly these frequent feeds will last for less than a week. You could ask the parents if their babies have grown out of their baby clothes! These appetite spurts often happen at 3 weeks, 6 weeks and 3 months and at 4 months. Parents may need extra support and reassurance from health visitors about the adequacy of breastfeeding to meet their babies' needs. There is no evidence that adding formula milk will improve their sleeping patterns. This is normal behaviour and babies are taking more milk to give them energy to grow. Parents may find it helpful to talk to others and peer supporters can be particularly helpful and reassuring for them to hear how others have coped with these more challenging times.

Introducing solid foods

The recommendations from WHO[4] and NHS England[5] are that infants should be breastfed exclusively for the first 6 months. We are aware that in the UK many parents start introducing solid foods before this time, perhaps misinterpreting signs of dribbling and putting objects in their mouths, as signs of hunger. This is one of the factors that leads to us having the lowest exclusive breastfeeding rates in the world of 1–2% at 6 months, although the infant feeding survey in 2010 showed that 34% of mothers are still breastfeeding at this time. Babies have immature digestive systems and are not ready to digest solids before 6 months.

The perceptions and practices around introducing solid foods to babies have followed a similar path to those relating to breastfeeding. In the 1970s solids foods were started early, around 3–4 months, and these were usually soft purees which were spoon fed. Babies of this age were unable to chew, so foods had to be made liquid enough to swallow. Dried foods which contained large numbers of additives became popular for their convenience and needed to be reconstituted with water. They were certainly nothing like real family foods! Lumpy foods were considered unsafe for small babies, and baby rice mixed with formula milk was often used but did not introduce babies to the tastes of family food.

Baby foods became commercialised and advertised in a similar way to formula milk but were not restrained by the International WHO Code and some foods still continue to be advertised as suitable for babies from 4 months, although this goes against the recommendations to breastfeed exclusively until 6 months. Health visitors in the 1960s to 1980s received free samples of these highly processed dried foods, to give to mothers, and we became unpaid promoters of these products. Parents thought they were giving their children modern, healthy nutrition and became reliant on these poor quality, expensive foods, rather than using their own family foods. Many children grew up without tasting fresh foods which may have contributed to the obesity epidemic we now have in the UK.

The research around introducing solid foods has not been extensive, although work by Gill Rapley[6] (a former health visitor) on baby-led weaning has shown that babies have behaviour and development at 6 months that makes them capable of independent eating, leading to them understanding and enjoying independent eating of healthy family foods. This way of introducing solid foods is becoming more mainstream around the world. There is also some evidence that introducing solids while breastfeeding helps babies progress more quickly, especially if given those that the mother eats. It is thought that breastmilk has some flavours from her diet, so these are familiar and more acceptable to her baby.[7] Children who were breastfed appear to choose a diet of healthy foods and are less likely to become obese.[8]

Babies' weight gain may slow as they transition on to eating solid foods and this should not be of concern, as milk is their main source of nutrition in the first year. Some are slow to accept new tastes and textures and it takes time for them to adjust to chewing, moving food boluses backwards in their mouths and swallowing them. Usually they know what their bodies need and, especially when solids are introduced in a baby-led way, will start to enjoy eating.

What will baby clinics look like after the pandemic?

The future looks uncertain for face-to-face contacts and at present it seems unlikely that baby clinics will return to their pre-pandemic style, certainly in the next few years, as mothers may be anxious to be bringing their babies to mix with large numbers of parents and children.

We all know some parents who come to clinic often may weigh their babies far too frequently and are scrutinising them intently. When babies are seen to be gaining weight in a linear way on their centile (after initially moving up or down in the early weeks) on the WHO centile weight chart, you can reassure them that their babies are feeding effectively. As we hopefully approach 'post-COVID' time and a 'new normal', we will need the other methods, suggested above, of assessing growth rather than the old reliance on scales.

Breastfeeding is the physiological norm[9]

Women's bodies are designed to feed their babies and breastfeeding can be thought of as the fourth trimester of pregnancy. Our babies are born immature and require the immunological protection of colostrum and breastmilk. As healthcare professionals, we have a responsibility to give optimum support to all parents who wish to do so. Babies are individuals and their weight gains will vary, so we need to guard against suggesting any supplements which could interfere with the supply of breastmilk available to them, leading to parents losing confidence in exclusive breastfeeding, which will give babies the maximum benefits and lifelong health.

Notes

1 National Institute for Health and Care Excellence (NICE) (2017) *Faltering Growth: Recognition and Management of Faltering Growth in Children.* Available at: www.nice.org.uk/guidance/ng75

2 NICE (2021) *Postnatal Care. Guidance.* Available at: www.nice.org.uk/guidance/ng194

3 Ibid.

4 WHO (2020) *Infant and Young Child Feeding.* Available at: www.who.int/news-room/fact-sheets/detail/infant-and-young-child-feeding

5 NHS (2020) *Our Baby's First Solid Foods.* Available at: www.nhs.uk/conditions/baby/weaning-and-feeding/babys-first-solid-foods/

6 Rapley, G. and Murkett, T. (2008) *Baby-led Weaning: Helping Your Baby to Love Good Food.* London: Vermillion.

7 Hausner, H. *et al.* (2010) 'Breastfeeding facilitates acceptance of a novel dietary flavour compound', *Clinical Nutrition (Edinburgh, Scotland)*, 29(1), pp. 141–148.

8 Rito, A. I. *et al.* (2019) 'Association between characteristics at birth, breastfeeding and obesity in 22 countries: The WHO European Childhood Obesity Surveillance Initiative – COSI 2015/2017', *Obesity Facts*, 12(2), pp. 226–243.

9 NICE (2017) *Faltering Growth: Recognition and Management of Faltering Growth in Children. Guidance.* Available at: www.nice.org.uk/guidance/ng75

9 Special situations, when breastfeeding might be more difficult

There are certain situations which might make breastfeeding more difficult to establish, especially in the early weeks. When babies or mothers have physical conditions, they may need extra or specialist support to build their milk supplies to establish a feeding pattern. When parents know they or their babies have certain conditions diagnosed in pregnancy, such as the need for premature delivery, multiple births or congenital anomalies, they can make plans with you to make their breastfeeding journeys easier.

In this chapter, I will look at different special situations which may make initiating and establishing breastfeeding more challenging. I have used mothers' words which I think will give us insight into their lived experiences. I include the words of a peer supporter and a specialist health visitor who share their experiences of supporting mothers in different situations. I will also include some practical suggestions in bullet points which may help you make breastfeeding plans with parents antenatally.

I will also consider the difficult living conditions experienced by mothers who find themselves in homeless accommodation or women's refuges when pregnant or have new-born babies and discuss whether breastfeeding is feasible when their lives are in turmoil.

How can mothers establish breastfeeding during the time their babies are in neonatal units?

Some new-born babies may spend time in neonatal units which can be challenging for parents, because they are separated emotionally and physically from them. Some of these babies may be premature and others may have other medical conditions. Breast-milk will give them huge benefits, as it is easily absorbed by their immature gut and will give them protection from infection and help to prevent necrotising enterocolitis (NEC). These babies will benefit from the immunity that breastfeeding can give them as they are more vulnerable to infection when they are preterm or small.

The separation of parents from their babies admitted to neonatal units has a profound emotional impact on them and disrupts the relationship-building process, as well as the beginning of breastfeeding. Many late preterm babies, who in the past would have been in special care units, are now cared for in transitional care areas,which means they can stay with their mothers and be breastfed when strong enough. These are often either in postnatal wards or near them so neonatal nurses and midwives can work together to care for the mother and baby. This arrangement benefits the breast-feeding dyad, as they can have skin-to-skin contact, touch, hear and smell each other, which stimulates their instinctive behaviour.

DOI: 10.4324/9781003139775-9

Mothers are usually encouraged to express their milk, even if babies are beginning to latch on the breasts, because at first they may tire more easily. Expressing is usually easier when they are close to their babies, as oxytocin (the love hormone) surges more readily and helps with 'letting down' their milk. In response to parents' touch, babies also make oxytocin which helps them begin to build their close attachment to them, as their needs for comfort, familiar sounds, smells and food are being met.

The following are some pointers which may help mothers establish their milk supplies if they are separated from their babies or they have been born very small:

- Try to have some skin-to-skin contact immediately after birth, if the baby is stable.
- Begin hand-expressing colostrum and collect with a syringe, as soon as possible after the birth.
- Spend as much time as they can in the unit with their babies.
- Express frequently, at least every 2–3 hours by hand.
- Use a hospital grade, double pump once hand-expressing 10ml or more at a feed.
- Continue to use a combination of hand and pump expressions to stimulate as much colostrum/breastmilk as possible.
- Try to do 'kangaroo care', which is continuous skin-to-skin, when the baby is medically stable.
- Investigate the availability and use of donor breastmilk in the unit.
- Try to have as much physical and verbal contact with the baby by stroking and talking.
- Watch the Baby Buddy app to see the sections on parent-centred care for babies in intensive/special care and how to express breastmilk.[1]
- Connect with the infant feeding lead/nursery nurses/peer supporters who may be available in the unit.
- Talk to other mothers in the expressing room!
- Hire a hospital grade, double electric breast pump when discharged and continue to express at least eight times in 24 hours.
- Look at a photo of the baby, relax, listen to music, think milk and compress the breasts while expressing – it helps the milk flow!
- Read any BLISS information on feeding and caring for a preterm baby.
- Familiarise your baby with your breasts, so she can smell and lick colostrum.
- Ask for help from an experienced lactation nurse, midwife or lactation consultant with attaching your baby on the breast, when baby is strong enough (see Figure 9.1).

A mother's story of breastfeeding a very premature baby

I had a trouble-free pregnancy with my son T, until a sudden diagnosis of intrauterine growth restriction (IUGR) at 26 weeks. It became apparent that T would have to be born within a few days to give him a chance of survival, and he was born by planned caesarean at 27 weeks exactly. I had always intended to breastfeed but assumed this would not be possible now, like my planned birth centre water birth. However, the neonatal doctors who prepared us for what to expect explained that my milk was so important for T that it would be considered part of his medical treatment. I was given a Bliss booklet about expressing and breastfeeding and there was a story in it by a mum who had breastfed her 25-week baby. I decided then that I was determined to breastfeed T in the longer term.

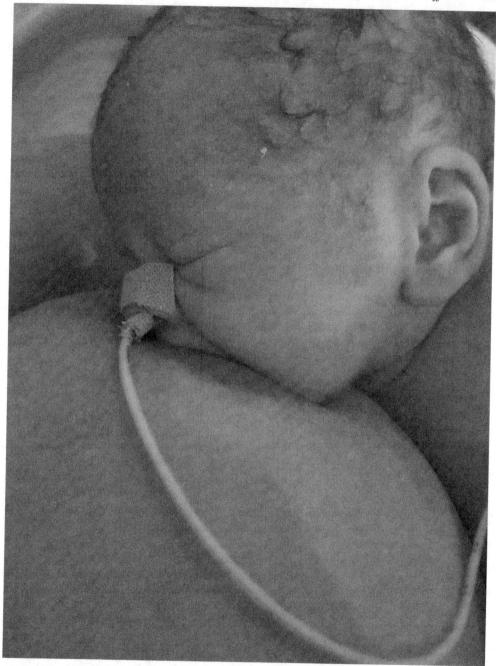

Figure 9.1 A premature baby beautifully latched

I began hand-expressing with little guidance and proudly produced 0.5ml colostrum the first time I tried. T was too sick to be fed at the start so everything I produced was carefully stored away. After a few days I was shown how to use a pump and the expressing room at the hospital became very familiar. Three at a time we would sit in there pumping, talking about our babies and swapping tips on how to get more milk.

T started on 0.5ml each four hours so I did not need to provide much milk at first, but I struggled to produce a full supply. After a few weeks I was prescribed domperidone on the advice of the nurses. This was very useful to me but looking back there was a lot I didn't know about expressing (such as power pumping) which could also have increased my supply. Pumping round the clock became part of daily life. After a very rough start when we thought we would lose him, T stabilised and made painfully slow progress as the weeks passed. This was a difficult, lonely time and the days were long.

Once T was term, I asked about feeding him directly. He was still on respiratory support and there wasn't much encouragement at first. Finally, a wonderful breastfeeding specialist nurse helped me to latch him on. We were lucky that he took to breastfeeding straightaway. Over the next couple of weeks, we developed a routine where I would feed him responsively in the daytime when I could be there. I came under some pressure to give bottles overnight. I never wanted to do this, but in the end, I agreed, and again I was lucky that T managed fine switching between bottle and breast.

My body responded to my baby as it had not to the pump and I finally produced milk in abundance. T was transferred for surgery around this time aged 4 months, and I recall the admitting doctor's 'wow!' on being told he had never had any formula. T was discharged on oxygen exclusively breastfeeding aged 5 months.

Breastfeeding T is the proudest achievement of my life. It was incredibly important for me to be able to do it after I had been unable to nurture him in the womb. It was also healing to our relationship, after such a difficult start, in ways that are hard to express. It was what really made me feel like his mother.

Can mothers exclusively breastfeed twins or multiple babies?

Antenatal contact

Antenatal contact provides an opportunity for community practitioners to have discussions with expectant parents to explore their feeding intentions. They also provide times to talk about the benefits of breastfeeding and strategies for feeding more than one baby in the early days. which may help parents become more confident about their abilities to breastfeed their babies for as long as they wish (Figure 9.2).

You could offer support by including the following information in this contact:

- Listen to their feelings and any previous experiences of infant feeding.
- Reassure mothers and their partners that exclusive breastfeeding twins or more, is possible, can save time, but may take time to establish in the early days.
- Explain about the production of colostrum from 18–20 weeks of pregnancy and encourage them to collect colostrum from 36 weeks, by hand-expressing into oral syringes and then freezing it.
- Give information about local antenatal breastfeeding workshops that mothers and partners can attend to learn about positioning and attachment of babies to gain good milk transfer.
- Explain why hand-expression before and after the births can help with stimulating their milk supplies.
- Discuss with parents that twins or triplets may encounter some issues, which can affect breastfeeding such as: they may be born early, are more likely to develop

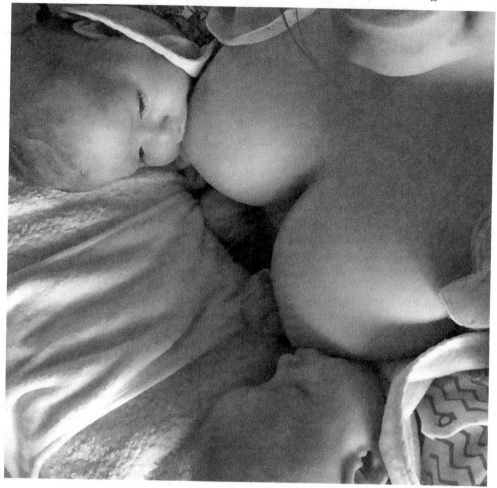

Figure 9.2 Twins tandem breastfeeding

jaundice, have low blood sugar and be receiving supplementation of infant formula when discharged from hospital.

- Signpost parents to their local twins' club, so they can talk to other mothers who have breastfed twins or more.
- Discuss online support and offer them the link below.
- Breastfeeding Twins and Triplets UK is a Facebook group for parents in the UK and Ireland, for twin and triplet families wishing to receive evidenced-based support to give them confidence to breastfeed their babies.[2]

After the births

At postnatal contacts, community practitioners have opportunities at their first new baby visit and subsequent contacts to support families of multiples with breastfeeding. There are a number of challenges that mothers may encounter, which may be helpful to understand. The following points could help you in your discussion with parents who wish to breastfeed multiple infants:

- Explain how skin-to-skin contact with mother can help babies elicit instinctive feeding behaviours and help them latch on the breasts.
- Discuss how fathers and partners can enjoy skin-to-skin too, which may calm the babies and at the same time, help them build close relationships with them.
- Describe babies' early feeding cues, which can help parents develop awareness of when their babies want to feed, rather than waiting for later cues such as crying.
- Explain the value of offering early, frequent breastfeeds and waking babies if sleepy.
- Discuss why early term and late preterm babies are more likely to be sleepy and may have feeding difficulties in the early weeks due to their age and developmental maturity.
- Observe both babies breastfeeding, if possible. Suggest adjustments to positioning and attaching their babies effectively and how to recognise when they are achieving good milk transfers with deep, long sucking bursts and swallowing, with pauses in between.
- Explain why feeding both babies at the same time, known as tandem feeding, will save parents time and will enable the slower feeder to benefit from the let down stimulated by the other baby, so will have a better flow of milk. One baby will need to be woken for a feed after the first one wakes, so both can be attached together.
- Share with parents what to look out for in babies' nappies to inform them about their milk intake.
- Explain the value of hand expressing/ pumping after feeds when possible, so that expressed milk can be given to babies, if they are sleepy or finding it difficult to achieve good milk transfer.
- Highlight that breast compressions can help, if babies are well attached, but not swallowing. Breast compressions involve mothers putting their hands in a C shape at the back of their breasts and squeezing their breasts gently for a few seconds.[3]
- If babies continue to be sleepy, use a hospital grade, double breast pump after every feed, if possible (These pumps can be hired from the main companies).
- Discuss the possibility of exclusive breastfeeding when infants are currently receiving breastmilk and supplementing with infant formula, if this is what parents wish.
- Vitamin D supplements (8.5–10mcg) are recommended for all exclusively breastfed babies from birth and for babies receiving less than 500mls of formula. Free Healthy Start vitamins are available for families who meet the criteria.

A mother's story of breastfeeding twins

When I found out I was expecting twins one of the first things I wondered was whether it was possible to breastfeed. Once the initial shock had worn off and I stopped being quite so sick I did some reading. This gave me the understanding that if my babies breastfed well and frequently, my breasts should respond by making the milk they needed. Twice the babies meant twice the stimulation which meant twice the milk. I was very lucky that my babies were born full term and healthy and they both latched on immediately. It was at this point I thought, 'Well if they can do it, I have to do it'. It was not an easy thing to do, but having twins, however you feed them, is not an easy thing to do! Several things made a big difference to our breastfeeding journey.

A midwife in the hospital showed me how to tandem feed on day 2. This was a game changer and I tandem fed pretty much every feed from then onwards. Once discharged, my community midwife helped me adjust the latch as I was getting quite sore. She also said I was doing brilliantly and also told me about the new breastfeeding group that was opening locally in a couple of weeks and that I should try to go. So, when the babies were 3 weeks myself and my partner walked to the breastfeeding café and received a very warm welcome. I now had somewhere I could go and get support, ask questions and chat to other mums. My other source of support was the local twins club. Only another mum of twins truly understands the difficulties. It was a lifesaver. Once breastfeeding was established, it was actually very easy and I think it really helped me cope with being a twin parent. Their milk was ready on tap, it helped them settle to sleep and there was no washing or sterilising. Also, I couldn't forget my boobs when I went out, I found my brain was not the most organised during the post-partum period! I also found it meant I could be the responsive parent that I wanted to be relatively easily, and I think it really protected our bond.

Insights found from parents' experiences from the Breastfeeding Twins and Multiples online support group[4]

- Twins and triplets are often born premature or early.
- Babies who were born a bit early often have a bit of a fussy period and feeding frenzy around 40-week gestation, as they move from early baby behaviour when they are sleepy, into full term new-born behaviour.
- Preterm babies often have fussy periods, growth spurts and developmental leaps at similar times to full term babies, which seem to be between actual age and adjusted age. Just because two babies are born on the same day, they do not always have their fussy periods at the same time.
- Personality plays a big part. One twin often needs more attention than the other, which makes parents feeling guilty about not cuddling their more independent sibling as much.
- Online support can enable many twins and more to exclusively breastfeed, even when they begin their breastfeeding journey with mixed feeding.
- Mothers report increased confidence in breastfeeding.

How peer support can help parents breastfeed twins.

A breastfeeding peer supporter, who had breastfed twins herself, reflects on her experiences of supporting parents with twins:

How peer support can help parents breastfeed twins

Kathryn Stagg, a breastfeeding peer supporter, who has breastfed twins herself, and specialises in supporting mothers with feeding twins and multiples, reflects on her experiences:

Many twins are born between 36 and 38 weeks gestation and this actually causes more difficulties than the fact that there are two babies to feed. Babies of this gestation are often sleepy and inefficient on the breast and so may need some additional milk in the early days. Again it can take time to establish breastfeeding, but once babies are strong enough to fully breastfeed, any top ups can be gradually stopped. During the early weeks parents again need lots of support with making sure the babies are latching well and feeding as efficiently as they can.

The role of peer support through this period is vital. For parents to be in a community, either online or face to face, where others have been through these journeys of initiating breastfeeding in premature or early term babies and come out the other side, breastfeeding is incredibly motivating. And the parents who are in the thick of it can see there is light at the end of the tunnel and it will get easier. As a breastfeeding supporter I love it if I can have continuity throughout their journey: so, firstly meeting them in the ante-natal period to discuss what to expect in different scenarios, again either in person or online, and then supporting them postnatally through the early stages until they are confident with latching, their ability to provide enough milk for their babies and understanding baby behaviour and responsive parenting. It is great when they are a couple of months down the line and everything is working well and the parents are achieving their goal.

The effectiveness of the peer support programme is due to the empathic relationship they have with the other women. There is a deep understanding of the other's situation within an equal power-relationship. The more we understand of oxytocin, one of the breastfeeding hormones, is that it is inhibited by the stress hormone cortisol, and released in situations of relaxation, love and trust.

Can babies with congenital heart disease breastfeed?

Parents will usually know from scans done in early pregnancy whether their babies have heart anomalies, which means they can make plans on how they wish to feed their babies. During your antenatal contact, you could discuss with them how breastmilk will help support their baby's immune systems, so reducing infections, while giving them easily absorbed, perfect nutrition. Initially mothers may need to express their breastmilk, but they could have skin-to-skin contact when their babies are medically stable and when they are strong enough, they can begin to breastfeed directly. This close contact helps mothers with their breastmilk supply and helps them build close, reciprocal loving relationships.

An interesting unpublished, MSc qualitative study was carried out at a paediatric cardiac centre in London a few years ago, where parents and staff were interviewed on film, and spoke about their experiences of caring for babies with cardiac conditions. A thematic analysis revealed that parents asked for tailored support for their own well-being and staff needed training in practical skills to support breastfeeding and communication skills. It was found that families' journeys can be challenging when establishing milk supplies and helping their babies feed directly from the breast, and parents wanted support at each stage. They asked to be involved in all staff discussions about feeding and identified the handovers between staff going through shift changes as very important.

Events in this study were organised when parents and staff met, and parents talked about the support and care needed when breastfeeding their babies with cardiac problems. Some babies required surgery and were not strong enough to breastfeed for a few days or weeks, depending on the severity of their condition. After this study, staff became more aware of the support parents needed and were more prepared to listen to their stories and focus on their emotional well-being.

There are some practical points which may be worth considering when supporting parents who have babies with cardiac problems:

- Antenatal hand-expression of colostrum from 36 week's gestation which can be stored in syringes in a freezer.
- After the birth, hand-expressing (8–10 times a day) even if the baby is beginning to attach to the breast, because he may tire quickly and this colostrum can be given directly to him.
- Skin-to-skin contact with parents is invaluable, when they can talk to their babies and stroke them, helping them build close, loving relationships. It will reduce their stress, by increasing oxytocin levels, boost babies' emotional brain development and reduce their pain when going through invasive procedures.
- Hospital grade, double breast pumps can be used to express, once frequent hand-expressions are resulting in larger volumes of colostrum. Expressing is best done next to their babies, but pumps can be hired for use at home, from the main breast pump manufacturers. Breast compressions while expressing can help more milk flow.
- Colostrum/breastmilk can be stored in a domestic fridge for five days, or a freezer for five months.
- Establishing a good milk supply in the first weeks will enable mothers to sustain breastfeeding for longer.
- Positioning and attaching babies on the breast will be easier once they become stronger and often easier when parents are more relaxed at home.
- Emotional support, listening to parents' stories and keeping in touch with them will help their breastfeeding journey.

A mother's story of breastfeeding her baby who had heart surgery soon after birth

I had planned to breastfeed my son, A, for as long as I could, knowing the benefits that this would have for him. However, I knew it would not be easy (or even possible) in our case. Thirteen weeks into the pregnancy, A was diagnosed with a congenital heart condition called Transposition of the Great Arteries. Very early on, I had to let go of the birth and new-born story that I had imagined because it was likely to be a very different experience for us. Because of his condition, the standard treatment protocol was to immediately take him away for life-saving treatment. There would be no skin-to-skin, no baby brought to my breast for his first feed, no proud mum and dad photos post-birth. The doctors weren't even sure whether I would get to properly see him.

Fortunately, A was born in a much better state than the doctors had expected and I was able to hold him for a few minutes until they cut the cord. I cried the whole time – overwhelmed with both relief and gratitude. But I will never forget that special moment. I didn't see him again until the following afternoon.

That night, in hospital, I learnt to hand-express my colostrum, supported by a wonderful team of midwives. The liquid was stored away in a tiny syringe. I remember feeling so excited to have filled a 1ml tube! It felt good to know there was something important I could do to help my baby – despite being apart. When we were finally reunited, 24 hours later, I was able to hand-feed him from the syringe. Again, not the experience we had expected but I was so grateful to have the opportunity to support him in this way.

In the days leading up to A's arterial switch (the operation that would save his life), I put myself on a strict expressing regimen. Every three hours, I set myself up for 15+ minutes of expressing. The cold, impersonal activity was a struggle particularly at night, given the physical and mental condition I was in. But I kept at it. Soon, I graduated from syringes to an electronic double pump. 1ml turned to 100ml quickly.

Initially we fed A the milk through a syringe or feeding tube, but by day 7 we had started to offer him a bottle. Whilst we had made an attempt to breastfeed during this time, it had proved too stressful. There was one particular moment I remember where I had A on my chest, trying to get him into the right position. On one side, I had a somewhat overbearing but well-intentioned lactation consultant trying to manoeuvre us both. On the other side, I had a nurse and my husband looking on, offering advice and reassurance. Both A and I were crying. Milk was leaking everywhere and we were tangled in medical cords and other equipment. I felt like such a failure. Why did it all have to be so hard? I was overwhelmed with love and terror in equal measure.

A week later, A had his open-heart surgery. I was terrified watching his tiny body wheeled away in an enormous bed. But I was proud to say that he was already back at his birth weight of 3.5kg by this stage. I hoped that that would count for something. He seemed strong too. A fighter already.

A spent six more weeks in hospital, four of them in the PICU. A series of complications during and post-surgery resulted in necrotising enterocolitis or deadening of the bowel. The treatment was antibiotics and fasting. We were devastated. But again, I focused on what I could control – expressing, expressing and more expressing. By this stage, I was only waking once through the night though as I felt emotionally drained from the tough days we were having. I knew I needed to keep myself going and that meant sleep.

I stored my milk in bags, froze them, and transported them to the hospital weekly in preparation for his recovery. There were some tough days there but eventually he turned the corner and it was time to start feeding him again. The milk was fed to him through a nasal gastric tube but we didn't care – this felt like a victory! Gradually (again), we went from 1ml to 10 to 20 to 160ml. He was suddenly feeding like a champ. All of the milk I had stored was used and then some formula. I tried to step up my expressing routine again but it was challenging, especially as I was doing it from a cold hospital room or at home, without my baby in my arms. Videos helped. I also tried breastfeeding teas and other supplements.

At around week 5, A graduated from the PICU into the regular children's ward and it was time to try breastfeeding again. The lactation consultant (LC) was optimistic that, given his impressive appetite pre-surgery, that he may be able to feed again although, with heart babies, this is often not a possibility. Unfortunately, it didn't work for us again and we had many challenging moments (i.e. eyes and nipples leaking simultaneously). My husband tried to help, as did the staff – not one but two LC's! The skin-to-skin boosted my supply so that was a plus but we just couldn't seem to get in sync.

It wasn't until we got home (week 7) that we found our groove. Sitting on my own couch, without the machines and bright lights. Suddenly, he latched! I couldn't believe it. All of the hard work had been worth it.

It wasn't all downhill from there though. During his illness, and associated fasting, A had lost a significant amount of weight in hospital. To assist weight gain, we were required to fortify my breastmilk with formula. Unfortunately, with our tough start, my supply was never quite able to keep up with his needs. After a week or so at home we chose to mix feed. At first this was probably 80/20 breastmilk to formula but over time, this shifted to 60/40. I was disappointed not to be able to exclusively breastfeed him especially given what he had been through. However, I was also incredibly grateful to be able to feed him at all. I maintained this routine for about ten months and then moved exclusively to formula. I cherished those many hours we spent together, breastfeeding, skin-to-skin after all of our time apart. Looking back, I have no doubt it benefited our relationship, as well as his health. Whilst those early days expressing were some of the hardest I can remember, I would do it all again in a heartbeat for the benefits I know it has given him.

Can mothers breastfeed their babies with Down Syndrome?

Breastfeeding can offer babies with Down Syndrome so many benefits, especially by helping their immune systems, leading to fewer or less severe infections, reducing allergies, asthma and obesity later in childhood. The act of drawing milk from the breast with their jaws will strengthen their facial muscles and tongues and help with future speech development. Babies with this condition may also have cardiac problems, so the points above may be useful here too. Parents may have been given this diagnosis in early pregnancy, so are able to plan and think about how they wish to feed their baby. If they decide to breastfeed, you can give them information on 'harvesting colostrum' from 36 week's gestation, which will help them learn this skill before the birth and have a supply to offer their babies, if they are too sleepy to breastfeed. Occasionally babies are not diagnosed until after the birth and parents may be feeling confused and unprepared.

Some babies with Down Syndrome will latch on their mothers' breasts in skin-to-skin soon after being born and have enough muscle strength to continue to breastfeed later, achieving good milk transfer and gaining weight. Other babies may find it harder to latch and breastfeed effectively because of low muscle tone and poor suck, swallow and breath coordination. Their parents may need more support in building and maintaining their breastmilk supply and feeding this to their babies.

The following points may be helpful in your antenatal and postnatal discussions:

- Signpost them to the local infant feeding support team, so they could visit existing groups run either by the NHS, or one of the third sector organisations (see list at the end of the book).
- Encourage antenatal expression of colostrum from 36 weeks which can be stored in a freezer.
- Offer emotional support antenatally and listen to parents' hopes and fears for their babies.
- Listen to their stories around the birth postnatally and how they are adjusting to life with their new babies, who may be facing challenges.
- Observe a feed to establish effective positioning, attachment and effective milk transfer.
- Offer information and support with expressing milk if their baby's suck is weak and explain that their baby may get stronger over time.
- Explain that the 'dancer hand position' can help to keep the baby's head steady while breastfeeding. The mother can hold under her breast with three fingers, with her thumb and index free to support the cheeks forming a U shape with the baby's chin resting in the bottom of the U. This helps to support the chin, so baby can maintain the latch.

- Monitor baby's weight gain on the green Down Syndrome growth chart, as weight gain may be slower.
- Mixed feeding with breastmilk and formula may be the way some parents decide to feed. Any breastmilk will provide some benefits to the baby.

The following helpful quote can be found on the Breastfeeding Network (BfN) website:[5]

> There are so many benefits in breastfeeding and these can apply even more so to babies with Down Syndrome. Breastmilk can boost your baby's immune system and provide protection against numerous auto-immune disorders such as coeliac disease, allergies and asthma to name a few. The act of breastfeeding itself will strengthen your baby's tongue, lips and face which helps with future speech development.
>
> Sadly, there is a myth that babies with Down Syndrome cannot breastfeed and I've heard many stories of mums not being supported or being told their baby won't breastfeed so not to bother trying by various healthcare professionals.
>
> Whilst it's absolutely possible for many babies with Down Syndrome to breastfeed efficiently and successfully, there are some factors that may arise which can impact on establishing feeding. Medical complexities, low muscle tone and lack of suck, swallow, breathe co-ordination are some of the additional challenges facing babies with Down Syndrome. As a result some mums will breastfeed as well as giving expressed breast-milk from a bottle/tube and others will move onto formula milk.[6]

Can mothers breastfeed when they have babies with developmental delay?

Breastfeeding a baby who has severe developmental delay is likely to present some problems. If the baby has very poor muscle tone, then he may not be able to sustain a latch on the breast for long and expressing milk may be the parent's only option if they want to give their babies breastmilk. If you remember from previous chapters, mother's milk actually flows to the baby during 'let down' under the influence of oxytocin, so sometimes it is easier for a baby to breastfeed than it is to bottle feed. The special ingredients of breastmilk, especially the immunity it confers, are especially important for these babies, so parents may ask you for support in either breastfeeding directly or expressing and storing breastmilk. The bullet points listed above may be helpful to consider in your discussions with parents. The 'dancer hand position' may be particularly helpful when attaching the baby to the breast.

Can babies with cleft lip and palate breastfeed?

Breastfeeding can be possible with both cleft lips and palates depending on their severity but mothers may be able to feed some expressed milk initially. Parents often need skilled help with positioning and attaching their babies, because they may take time to form a seal with their mouths on the breasts. There are many advantages for the baby in having breastmilk because it helps to give protection against infections, especially those of the ear, and the action of the baby's jaws will help to strengthen the facial and mouth muscles. Breastmilk also does not irritate the delicate tissue in the nose and throat in the way that formula does. Parents need to be prepared for some leakage of milk through the nose, which may alarm them but does no harm to the baby.

Cleft lips and palates are the most common craniofacial abnormality in the UK, affecting 1 in 700 children, that is 1,200 babies a year. A cleft lip is when the tissue which makes up the lip does not join properly in pregnancy, resulting in an opening in the upper lip. This can be small or extend into the nose and is usually corrected surgically when the baby is between 3 and 6 months old. A cleft palate is where the roof of the mouth has not joined and can affect the hard or soft palate, which can be repaired usually when the baby is 6 to 12 months old.

Sometimes these two conditions are associated with a syndrome called Pierre Robin Sequence, which is a set of abnormalities affecting the face, lower jaw and tongue. Diagnosis of these abnormalities may be made through scans before birth or during the new baby paediatric examination.[7] Referral to a multidisciplinary, specialist team can be made, and a feeding care plan started, before the baby is discharged from hospital. Parents often find it helpful to talk to other parents about their experiences, through organisations such as CLAPA, so they can be reassured of the successful results of surgery.[8]

You might find the following points helpful when giving parents information before the baby is born, adapting the information depending on the severity of the cleft lip or palate:

- Antenatal diagnosis will give the pregnant woman time to collect some colostrum if she wishes and freeze it in syringes.
- Skin-to-skin after birth will help with oxytocin release and bonding, but baby may find it hard to attach to the breast in this position.
- Start hand-expressing as soon as possible after the birth and continue every 2–3 hours and as colostrum/breastmilk volume increases use a hospital grade double pump 8–10 times a day.
- Nasogastric feeding may sometimes be necessary initially if the baby does not manage to attach to the breast or bottle.
- Ask for skilled help with positioning and attaching the baby on the breast.
- Try different positions but often ones where baby is upright stops milk leaking through the nose, if the baby has a cleft palate.
- Breasts are soft and flexible and can mould into the lip and mouth and make a seal.
- Mother can hold her breast with the 'dancer hand position', cupping her breasts with her hands in a C-shape and supporting the baby's jaw with a finger to steady it in her baby's mouth, so keeping her nipple at the back of his mouth.
- Breast compressions can help to move more milk to the baby.
- Continue to express milk until baby is breastfeeding effectively.
- Expressed milk can be given by a 'squeezable, specialist bottle' as advised by the specialist team.

How can milk banks help?

Human milk banks across the UK offer donated breastmilk to hospital neonatal units for small and sick babies. The Hearts Milk Bank[9] in the South East of England has its aim that all babies should have the opportunity to benefit from human milk and sometimes can be very helpful when babies or mothers are sick in the community and breastfeeding is not possible for a period of time. In Scotland and other areas in the

UK, some milk banks can supply donated breastmilk to mothers in some community settings and it is hoped that this provision can be expanded in the future. In all milk banks, the donors have their blood screened and their milk is tested to ensure safety and then frozen. If you see mothers who have more breastmilk than they need for their baby, you could suggest they donate to a milk bank. Many women are happy to express their milk once a day and freeze it, before it is collected from their home by the milk bank drivers.

There is debate at the moment in the EU as to whether breastmilk should be classified as a biofluid, because it contains human tissue and cells, rather than just a food which it is at the moment. There are some worrying trends for private companies in the UK and other countries, to commercialise donated breastmilk which are not regulated and do not conform with the NICE guidelines (2010).[10] Synthetic breastmilk is being manufactured in the US from human stem cells and the efficacy and safety of this has yet to be shown. Milk sharing has become more popular recently where some mothers may want to give their expressed milk to friends or family, but there is risk of passing on bacteria or viruses with this practice as the milk is not being tested. Any breastmilk sold on the Internet which comes from unknown, unregulated donors has not been microbiologically or content tested and cannot be trusted.

Can mothers breastfeed if they are unwell?

If mothers become unwell with viral or bacterial infections while they are breastfeeding, they may worry that they could pass them to their babies. You can reassure them that the best thing they can do for them is to continue to breastfeed because of the antibodies and anti-infective properties in their milk.

Mothers' milk contains antibodies or immunoglobulins from their blood, which they make in response to an infection. There are five basic types called IgG, IgA, IgM, IgD and IgE, which are all found in human milk, but the prominent form is secretory IgA, which is also found in the guts and respiratory systems of adults. The secretory component seems to shield the antibody from being destroyed by gastric juice and digestive enzymes in the stomach and intestines of the infant. When a mother inhales a pathogen, the lymph nodes in her lungs make specially sensitised lymphocytes that travel to her breasts where specific antibodies are made against that bacteria or virus, which then pass into her milk. Another mechanism is taking place which is only beginning to be understood, whereby if the baby's saliva contains any pathogens, messages are sent backwards in the breast during feeding to the lymphatic tissue to make antibodies. There are also phagocytes in the milk, which are white cells that kill bacteria and viruses by engulfing them. (This is why breastmilk can cure babies' or adults' eye or skin infections!)

If mothers are suffering from non-communicable diseases, such as diabetes, heart disease, mental health disorders, epilepsy, or inflammatory conditions, they may be concerned that they may affect their babies, or that drugs they take may not be compatible with breastfeeding. There are only a few drugs which are not suitable for breastfeeding mothers but there are usually alternative drugs which can be prescribed. Parents may also worry about alcohol intake, anaesthetics, hay fever medication, or hair dyes. For information on drugs in breastmilk you can suggest that they go to the Breastfeeding Network's (BfN) website, which has been written and is regularly updated by a specialist pharmacist.[11]

What if either mother or baby need to be hospitalised?

Breastfeeding can usually continue if babies are admitted to paediatric wards because most hospitals have policies that enable mothers to stay with them and breastmilk is likely to accelerate their recovery. If babies are so unwell or weak that they are unable to attach to their breasts, then breast pumps should be available for them to express their milk and give it to their babies, perhaps by nasogastric tubes.

If mothers have to be admitted to hospital because they are unwell or need an operation, they could ask for a single room, so their babies could stay with them to be breastfed. If they are too unwell to care for them, then fathers or other family members may need to take their babies home and feed them expressed milk, until their mothers are well enough to breastfeed. You may need to advocate for families with hospital staff and help them work out a plan, so that breastfeeding can continue once mothers are discharged.

How can we support mothers living in homeless hostels or refuges?

Mothers who live in homeless hostels or refuges are less likely to initiate or continue to breastfeed for 6 months. A large analysis across five low-income and middle-income countries showed that those who have been subjected to intimate partner violence are 12% less likely to initiate breastfeeding and 13% less likely to breastfeed exclusively for the first 6 months. Forty per cent of women exposed to violence in the past 12 months were likely to stop breastfeeding before 4 months, and women exposed to several types of abuse were 50% more likely to stop breastfeeding compared to women who had not been exposed to abuse.[12]

A large, prospective, cohort study in Norway also identified past and recent abuse of women as strongly associated with early cessation of breastfeeding.[13] They also found that women who had been exposed to sexual abuse as children were significantly more likely to stop breastfeeding before their babies reached 4 months old.

Another study in the USA suggested that there were ethnic differences in breast-feeding after domestic abuse. They found that white women who had been exposed to violence were more likely to stop breastfeeding early, but black women were more likely to make breastfeeding plans and continue for longer.[14]

My colleague, who is a specialist in the issues facing homeless families and women who have been subjected to domestic abuse told me:

> My personal experience has shown that within the homeless and refuge accom-modation there is a genuine honesty from people who don't understand anything about breastfeeding. First, infant feeding decisions seem to be made prior to, or irrespective of, direct contact with health professionals during pregnancy, child-birth or early motherhood.
>
> Whilst one might expect women suffering DVA to be less informed of the advantages of breastfeeding, to be more affected by feelings of disgust and embarrassment and to be more likely to formula feed, my professional experience cannot always support these conclusions. However, some tentative conclusions can be drawn that there are several factors which affect the initiation (and duration) of breastfeeding with this population. Breastfeeding was generally perceived as an activity which is 'out of place' in hostel and hotel settings, where the majority of

clients were formula feeding. They perceived breastfeeding to be embarrassing, disgusting and inconvenient, whilst at the same time acknowledging that 'breast is best'. Their behaviour is influenced by a wide range of personal, social, economic and cultural factors.

When I talk to my clients in homeless accommodation or in a refuge setting clients tell me that they just don't like the idea of it, that they are stressed, upset, desperate to manage their situations and all this not allowing them the time to breastfeed. I rattle off my long list of the benefits! Often with no effect. But, I have had some successes also.

These very vulnerable clients need very sensitive support to breastfeed, especially if they have been subjected to violence and sexual abuse and their lives are very complicated and their futures uncertain. They may think that this is not the *time* to breastfeed and that it is *out of place* (to use my colleague's words) in a hostel or refuge setting. This brings me back to the main themes of this book, that the *time* of women's lives and the *place* where they do it has to feel right, in order for breastfeeding to be acceptable and appropriate. Perhaps if community practitioners, midwives and GPs can identify these women in pregnancy, breastfeeding plans could be made with them, so extra support can be made available, ideally empathic peer support which can relate to their difficult situations, could enable them to gain the confidence to breastfeed.

In this chapter, I have used mothers' and practitioners' words to give us some understanding of parent's lived experiences and how they have overcome some of their difficulties to be able to give their babies this healthy start to their lives. They demonstrate how strong women are to be able to overcome these profound challenges. We need to respect them and with them plan any extra support they feel would be useful, to make their breastfeeding journeys easier, enabling them and their babies to enjoy the closeness and long-term health benefits.

Notes

1 Best Beginnings (2021) 'Baby Buddy App'. Available at: https://web.bestbeginnings.org.uk/web/videos/premature–sick-babies-small-wonders
2 See www.facebook.com/groups/bftwinsuk
3 See https://youtu.be/60R7pd-HCtE
4 See https://breastfeedingtwinsandtriplets.co.uk/
5 The Breastfeeding Network (2021, 21 March) *Breastfeeding and Down Syndrome: Information for Families & Breastfeeding Supporters.* Available at: www.breastfeedingnetwork.org.uk/breastfeeding-and-down-syndrome/
6 The Breastfeeding Network (2021) *Down's Syndrome and Breastfeeding.* Available at: www.breastfeedingnetwork.org.uk/downs-syndrome-and-breastfeeding/
7 The GP Infant Feeding Network (UK) (2019, 4 October) *Cleft Lip and Palate.* Available at: https://gpifn.org.uk/cleft/
8 Cleft Lip and Palate Association UK (CLAPA) (2021). Available at: www.clapa.com
9 Hearts Milk Bank (2020) *About Us – HMB.* Available at: https://heartsmilkbank.org/about-us
10 NICE (2010) *Donor Milk Banks: Service Operation.* Guidance. Available at: www.nice.org.uk/guidance/cg93
11 The Breastfeeding Network (n.d.) 'Drugs in breastmilk – Is it safe?' Available at: www.breastfeedingnetwork.org.uk/detailed-information/drugs-in-breastmilk/

12 Caleyachetty, R. *et al.* (2019) 'Maternal exposure to intimate partner violence and breast-feeding practices in 51 low-income and middle-income countries: A population-based cross-sectional study', *PLOS Medicine*, 16(10), p. e1002921.
13 Sørbø, M. F. *et al.* (2015) 'Past and recent abuse is associated with early cessation of breast feeding: results from a large prospective cohort in Norway', *BMJ open*, 5(12), p. e009240.
14 Holland, M. L. *et al.* (2018) 'Breastfeeding and exposure to past, current, and neighborhood violence', *Maternal and Child Health Journal*, 22(1), pp. 82–91.

10 Can anthropology give us insights into the way society views breastfeeding?

Anthropology can give us insights into breastfeeding as a complex process which is emmeshed in social, historical, political, economic and religious contexts. In many parts of the world it may be the only option for feeding babies, but as economic improvements in a country open up, the possibility of purchasing formula milk arises. In all societies decisions on infant feeding are made within families in their kin groups, and the focus rests on women's bodies where controls of its boundaries may be made. I decided to study this discipline at a postgraduate level to see if I could look at breastfeeding through a different lens and gain more in-depth knowledge of women's experiences and wider societal influences. I carried out my fieldwork in North London and India, using qualitative methods of participant observations, interviews and ethnography. In this chapter I will begin by looking at some theoretical underpinnings of the anthropology of the body and how they can help us understand women's bodies when breastfeeding. I will look at the place where women feel it is acceptable to breastfeed and the time controls society may place on them.

Is breastfeeding an individual woman's learned skill?

Bourdieu was a French sociologist/anthropologist/philosopher who wrote about the way society can become deposited in bodies of people, affecting how they think, feel and act in certain ways and I think his idea of 'habitus'[1] could be applied to breastfeeding. In this theory, he argues that human behaviours are influenced by society, rather than by individual action leading to behaviours which are enduring and transferable. They are created and reproduced unconsciously but are not fixed and can be changed over time through history.

Everyone has their own 'habitus' as a way of conducting or controlling their bodies. This is reproduced unconsciously, not fixed and can be changed with time through history. Bodily knowledge or 'habitus' can be seen in different 'fields' that are networks, structures or sets of relationships, that can be situated in intellectual, religious, educational and cultural arenas.

In the 'field' of breastfeeding, I would argue that 'habitus' can be seen in women's bodies by the way they behave when feeding their babies. Other women who have breastfed their own babies will convey their bodily 'habitus' that is positive towards breastfeeding, not only in what they say and communicate, but also in how they present their bodies. Women who have grown up in families or societies where breastfeeding was expected and normal are more likely to follow this behaviour when they give birth to their own children. These are not conscious actions, but embodied

DOI: 10.4324/9781003139775-10

behaviour and knowledge, which has been passed through generations, families and societies.

In Western societies, where many women grow up in families and communities where breastfeeding is not seen, it does not become part of a young girl's or woman's 'habitus' or bodily action. I would suggest that women who breastfeed or have breastfed carry this special knowledge and express it through their bodies. This may be the way breastfeeding peer supporters carry this skill and are able to support other women with their embodied gestures, which are communicated in an unconscious way. Once enough women in a community have received this 'habitus', they carry it with them into community settings such as cafés, schools, playgroups, offices and social gatherings, so making breastfeeding the accepted way to feed babies. In this way, it can become 'normalised' in a community and passed on to others over time.

Can breastfeeding help to reduce social inequalities?

Inequalities in health may not always follow economic deprivation. If we look at the UK situation, some geographical areas in the North of England have low rates of breastfeeding and also have low life expectancy and a higher burden of disease. Others, for example, in London, may have poor housing and low incomes but have high breastfeeding rates and potentially better health outcomes. Michael Marmot argues that: 'Social hierarchies and health are much more than income.'[2]

Bourdieu also argued that power is culturally and symbolically created, leading to 'social, cultural or symbolic capital'[3] which plays an important role in societal power relations. It provides the means for a non-economic form of domination and hierarchy to hide the causes of inequality, which can impact on the values and activities of everyday life. Societies that feel disempowered may make life choices which might inadvertently lead to the continuation of health inequalities. This could be applied when parents make choices about feeding babies which could lead to poorer health outcomes for them and the next generation.

These theories may seem rather complex at first, but give us a way of understanding how societal influences may act on women's bodies in an unconscious way; so when decisions are made to breastfeed, they may not be simple life-style choices, but a result of their embodied life experiences and those of their families and communities.

How can the focus on the body help us understand women's lived experiences?

Nancy Scheper-Hughes and Margaret Lock argued that the *'mindful, lived body'*[4] experience can communicate with others through social, cultural and political means. They suggested that a helpful way of looking at this was to divide the body into three aspects:

1   *The individual body* – an intuitive sense of being an embodied self; as an individual experiencing usual sensations such as tiredness, cold, hunger, thirst etc. and sense of self. Also, the sense of 'lived experience' where there is a difference between what is contained within our skin and outside it. How an individual's body is conceived is different between cultures.

2   *The social body* – a symbol of how we think and map our bodies into the social world and is a natural metaphor in much of our communications. It includes the

body in health and sickness. We speak of healthy and sick societies and cultures as if they were collective bodies.

3 *The body politic* – the political regulation, control and surveillance of the individual or the collective social body, in order to obtain collective order and stability.

Through considering these three bodies, it could help us understand the way we think about nature, society, cultural meanings and the interaction of bodies in their social worlds. This could be very helpful when we try to understand the bodies and lived experience of breastfeeding mothers.

Scheper-Hughes in her book *Death Without Weeping* describes how the availability and promotion of formula milk in Brazil led to mothers losing their traditional breastfeeding practice and start formula feeding, so reducing their milk supplies and increasing the risk of their children dying of malnutrition and disease. She looked at this situation through the impact this had on women's bodies and the social pressures it put on them. Women began to feel that they were feeding their babies the best milk and expected the babies' fathers to buy it for them, but because many of the families she studied were very poor, the milk was often watered down to make it go further, which led to babies dying of malnutrition. Over time, they began to lose confidence in the quality and quantity of their breastmilk, as their supplies reduced after the introduction of supplementary milks.

Impoverished Brazilian mothers saw breastmilk as 'sour, curdled, bitter and diseased,' a metaphorical projection of their inability to pass on anything untainted to their children. Scheper-Hughes argued that: 'The natural products of blood, milk, tears, semen and excreta may be used as a cognitive map to represent other natural, supernatural, social and even spatial relations.'[5]

Why does breastfeeding in public places remain a problem in the UK?

The Equality Act (2010)[6] states that breastfeeding mothers should not be prevented from feeding their babies in public places and that it is 'unlawful for a business to discriminate against a woman because she is breastfeeding a child'. Despite this legislation, parents are confused! They know that breastfeeding is the healthiest option but realise that many people in our society still have problems seeing it in cafés, parks, restaurants etc. so it tends to be hidden, with many new parents never having seen a baby breastfeeding when they have their first child. Some theories suggest this could be due to breasts being sexualised as attractive to men in Western countries, which is reinforced by images in magazines, films, on billboards and on the Internet, as highlighted by poet Hollie McNish in her book about becoming a new parent called *Nobody Told Me*. She describes the way she had to breastfeed her baby in the unhygienic toilets in cafés and restaurants because it was not acceptable to feed in front of others:

> I thought it was okay, I could understand the reasons,
> They said,
> 'There might be a man or a nervous child seeing this small piece of flesh that they weren't expecting'
> But when I'm told I'd be better just staying at home
> And when another friend

I know was thrown off a bus
And another mother told to get out of a pub
Even my grandma said that maybe I was sexing it up
And I'm sure the milk-makers love all this fuss
All the cussing, and worry, and looks of disgust
As another mother turns from nipples to powder
Ashamed or embarrassed by the comments around her
And as I hold her head up and pull my cardie across
And she sips on that liquor made from everyone's God.[7]

These graphic descriptions about Hollie's experiences as a new mother trying to breastfeed in public places in the UK underline the dilemmas faced by mothers. The ways that breasts are displayed as sex objects is likely to be one factor, but in my experience, it is not only men who object to seeing it, but often other women who police it, by objecting to mothers breastfeeding in public. In some parts of the world, breastfeeding is seen in villages, towns, streets, work- places, where breasts are not covered in way they are in European countries. It is interesting that Hollie and other mothers are asked to feed their babies in toilets, as if the act of breastfeeding was somehow like passing urine or stools and not the place you would think of eating your sandwich! I think anthropology of the body could give us some additional insights here, as to why these substances coming out of the body need to be hidden from the public gaze, as if they are in some way dangerous or polluting to others.

All cultures have unspoken rules determining how to control substances that come into and out of the body and the place where this is acceptable. Mary Douglas was an anthropologist who focussed on the body and its entrances and exits. She argued that societies will attempt to control the place where this is acceptable, in order to prevent pollution and any potential dangers that might arise if milk leaked out in the wrong place and wrote: 'The most dangerous pollution is for anything that has once emerged gaining re-entry.'[8]

Breastmilk could then be seen as needing to be controlled to avoid pollution and a danger to society, because of its status as a fluid which has exited from the mother's body and entered her baby's body. This may require even greater vigilance than those applied to controls over other body fluids, such as sperm, urine and stools. Mary Douglas identifies two bodies, the physical and the social and the continual exchange of meaning between the two; as a result, the body becomes a restricted medium of expression.

My research with Indian women in the UK showed that they are in a state of ritual impurity after childbirth:

> The exits from the woman's body in the form of blood or milk will also be regu-
> lated by sanctions being put in place where her physical body can reside. Her
> mother will suggest she stays in her bedroom for the first week until her blood flow
> reduces, so she does not pose a danger to others in the household.[9]

This insight on the potential posed by body fluids leaking out may throw light on why public breastfeeding is still be seen by some in UK society as taboo and potentially polluting and dangerous in uncontrolled places. It may explain why women feel they need to be discreet to protect themselves and others.

Is breastfeeding a rite of passage?

Anthropologists argue that during the immediate weeks after giving birth, women and their babies go through rites of passage as they move from their old to new states of becoming new mothers; and infants to independent, post-uterine life. At this time, both women and babies are thought to be vulnerable to evil attack, while they are *betwixt and between* these two states. These rites of passage are applied to the period after birth for mothers and babies, Van Gennep[10] first described how these rites of passage, with their accompanying rituals, follow clearly defined stages of separation; *the pre-liminal rites; liminal rites*; and *rites of re-aggregation* or *post-liminal*, as they transform to their new state. This way of analysing this time can aid our understanding of cultural beliefs around the vulnerability of parents and their new babies, requiring traditional rituals to protect them. Cultures may have specified lengths of times when protection during these liminal periods may be needed, but they commonly last for a month, or 40 days after the birth. Rituals may be done at the end of this time to mark the transformation into their new state, which may involve a visit to a temple, mosque, church or GP postnatal check!

Mary Douglas has suggested that dangers may be present while a person is changing from one status to the next:

> Danger lies in transitional states, simply because transition is neither one state nor the next, it is undefinable. The person who must pass from one to another is himself in danger and emanates danger to others. The danger is controlled by ritual which precisely separates him from his old status, segregates him for a time, and then publicly declares his entry to his new status.[11]

Are women vulnerable in their 'liminal time' after childbirth?

Anthropologists argue that when the mother is in this transitional, liminal time between pregnancy and motherhood, and her child between intrauterine life and independent living, this makes them both vulnerable to evil attack as their status is uncertain and they need to be protected by rituals. In my research in London and India I found that South Asian grandmothers usually perform these, by passing water over the children's heads seven times every day and tying black threads on the baby's wrists or waists, putting black spots around the child's eyes or soles of the feet. These are thought to protect the body boundaries from evil attack. The rituals carried out may be different in many ways, but all have similar aims to protect the body boundaries. These beliefs were prevalent in the UK and in India but only revealed to me once I had built up a trusting relationship with some of the women because it is something not usually spoken about. Here are some of the thoughts they shared:

> Because we have this thing about the evil eye, Asian women will not feed in front of other Asian women. They feel that the woman might cast an evil eye on the child, and then you will stop producing milk. They are cautious about who they feed in front of and will probably restrict it to just direct family. If there is someone else there, they will not come out and feed their child. It is not the shame of showing a boob, it is out of fear of casting the evil eye. She may be jealous and think, oh, she's got a beautiful baby, or she's having milk and I couldn't do it; or it

could be that she has a boy and I've got a girl, it could be a hundred and one things and she could come from the most modern families.[12]

There may be generational changes, but I found in my research that women in the UK were more likely to adhere to these beliefs than women in India.

There is a generation change. My mother-in-law believes in the evil eye more strongly than me. Older people believe that you have to pass a container of water, glass or steel, around the baby's head seven times in a clockwise direction. Then you take it outside the front door, not the back, to a crossroad and pour the water on the roads without looking at it.[13]

Another mother said:

My mother-in-law told me not to feed in front of anyone, because we don't want anyone casting an evil eye on him. I would have breastfed him if there were no other Asian mothers present. We do not think that white people have the same problem with jealousy.[14]

I found that older women in the household were likely to advise their daughters or daughters-in-law about where they could breastfeed. You may have also seen the way bottles of formula milk are covered up, so no jealous person can look at the milk with a jealous eye and make the baby unwell. Men in the household did not make any comments about controlling the place where their wives could feed.

Is there time for breastfeeding in the UK?

Breastfeeding occurs within this *liminal time* for mothers and their babies, happening between intrauterine life for the child and pregnancy and parenthood for the parents. As I described above, this can be a vulnerable time for both and they may need the protection of rituals.

Babies do not understand *clock time*! They follow their bodies' needs for nutrition, growth and comfort by giving their parents feeding cues, which tend to be frequent in the first few days and months. We live in *industrial time* in Europe, where almost everything we do and plan is based around the clock and *linear time*; but in other parts of the world people may follow the natural time of the sun and natural flows of rivers. Kahn has described lactation as part of the 'organic cycle of life', 'agricultural' or 'maialogical time'[15] but women in industrial societies may have lost touch with this closeness to their body rhythms in the UK. The word 'mai' is a Greek word meaning mother or nurse from the root 'ma' which is the sound of the child's cry for her mother. Kahn described her own experiences of breastfeeding:

After being at work, with deadlines, schedules and meetings, everything marked off by the clock, I would float with him into a different time. It was more cyclical, like the seasons, the tides, like milk which kept its own appointment with him, without me planning it out. I lived those years in two kinds of times-agricultural and industrial.[16]

Childcare manuals and experts in Western countries have recommended controls over breastfeeding by advocating strict time schedules such as 3-hourly feeds and length of feeds on both breasts, rather than trusting babies' feeding cues and their strong instincts to communicate these to their parents. Mothers who have come to the UK from India have told me that there was plenty of time to breastfeed there, even when they were working in fields, but after they moved to the UK, there was no time for breastfeeding. Linear, industrial time has made constraints on this natural body flow from mother to baby.

In my research with Indian mothers in the UK, many talked of the importance of 'milk flows':

> No matter how I tried to breastfeed here, the milk just didn't flow. I tried it for a week, and I got the feeling the child was hungry, because he used to take a lot of water from the bottle. I think it was my mother who said that you are not going to flow, the best thing to do is to put him on powered milk.

Another mother remembered breastfeeding when living in rural India:

> I liked working on the farm. We used to grow peanuts, potatoes and onions and used water from the well. I miss it – they had a much better life than here – they had freedom. If they have extra work, then they call other ladies to help. When we are breastfeeding, we are free from work. At night when babies wake up and are crying, we breastfeed in bed, it is hard to bottle feed.[17]

Why is the language of breastfeeding influenced by industry and Western medicine?

My research with Indian mothers suggested that the word 'breastfeeding' is a mechanistic term implying only the transfer of milk from a mother to her baby, where the focus is on the breast and the baby's mouth, not on mothers' and babies' bodies, emotions and minds. This separates their emotions, the nurturing element of the process and the natural and social world around them. I also found that the industrial metaphors, such as 'milk production' and 'supply and demand' that surround breastfeeding implied that the process is thought of as hard work for mothers and babies. The time restraints, such as '3-hourly feeding', '20 minutes a side in order to get to the hindmilk', do not allow for the reciprocity of breastfeeding, where mothers' bodies and emotions respond to their babies feeding, so they become united as dyads. These time constraints move women away from their bodily flows, which are embedded in their natural cycles of life.

These mechanical terms and the way breasts have been objectified only serve to distance women and their babies from their embodied experience of breastfeeding. Photographs and diagrams of disembodied breasts and babies' mouths, demonstrating the importance of attachment, are seen in medical and nursing textbooks, reinforcing that these body parts can almost be separated from whole bodies.

In 2006, Fiona Dykes used qualitative methods to do an ethnographic study of women's experiences of breastfeeding in a hospital in the UK and found that first-time mothers in particular frequently felt unsupported when they came to feed their babies. She found an impersonal, medicalised environment where midwives were overworked, leading to a situation where neither the service-user nor the provider of care felt satisfied. She likened it to a production line and also found that industrial time and metaphors regulated the natural behaviour of mothers and babies.[18]

Why has this natural process been medicalised?

The deep entrenchment of these mechanistic concepts in Western thought is demonstrated in the way that the biomedical system has tried to medicalise, manage, measure and control breastfeeding, rather than listening to and supporting mothers and babies in their social context. Through this process, women's bodies and emotions have become alienated and their breastmilk turned into a precious commodity that can be extracted from breasts. The cultural context of women's lives has been generally ignored, with hospitals and clinics reinforcing the need for correct breastfeeding techniques as the only answer for successful breastfeeding. The language of health professionals reinforces the power divide in their relationships with parents, rather than listening to their experiences and the social situations they inhabit. This may result in them losing their self-efficacy and relying on midwives, hospital doctors, health visitors and GPs for answers to their questions, rather than their own intuition or that of families and friends.

Many academics have written about the medicalisation of the natural act of breastfeeding, Penny Van Esterick pioneered the social science's research into breastfeeding which has subsequently widened and moved into many disciplines such as historical, feminist and critical medical anthropology. She was concerned about the way breastfeeding was being medicalised and said that: 'Medicalisation individualises human problems and removes them from their social and economic context.'[19]

Cecilia Tomori *et al.* examine new anthropological perspectives in their interesting book which argues that, although scientific evidence on breastfeeding has moved global public health to promote it with the aim of restoring it to the norm, this has led to policies and practices which promote the product breastmilk as the healthiest way to feed babies, but do not focus on the challenges faced by women. They quote Van Esterick here in her summing up some of the complexities of breastfeeding in bottle-feeding communities:

> Anthropology has the potential to make explicit the interconnectedness between social relations, resources, sexuality, embodiment, power, nurturance, and commensality implicated in the challenge of feeding a new-born infant. No other discipline is positioned to ask and answer such fundamental questions about what makes us human.[20]

Vanessa Maher in her excellent book on the anthropology of breastfeeding also suggests that:

> The medical model as regards breastfeeding appears to belong to an out-dated positivist system, which is anthropologically interesting but highly dangerous, if it is to inform policies towards women.[21]

Some Indian women I spoke to during my research were still connected with the natural, religious and traditional context of breastfeeding and told me:

> All animals have milk and it is natural to feed their young, so we should do it. It's nature's way of looking after the baby. You only have breastmilk after having a baby and you must feed your own milk, as God made it especially for your child.

> Breastfeeding your child is thought to be one of the best things you can do. It is part of your karma, or life force. If you breastfeed someone, you do them a very big favour.[22]

The older Indian women I spoke to also thought that breastfeeding was an important time for women to rest after childbirth. There was a feeling that new mothers were keen to continue their period of ritual impurity during this liminal time of 40 days after birth, when they do not work and are looked after by kin, so they can focus on feeding their babies. Rituals are done to protect both mothers and babies from any potential harm at this uncertain time. I was told that older women in India have cultural knowledge of breastfeeding and relied on their kin for support, not health professionals: 'My mother-in-law told me that breastfeeding is best for babies' health, so I breastfed my daughter for 2 years. She had breastfed her children for 4 years each. They all believe it is good.' [23]

Can mothers' emotions be transferred to babies during breastfeeding?

The close connection between mothers and babies when breastfeeding enables early relationship building between the two. The rise in the hormone oxytocin helps to cement this, not only between the two of them, but possibly within families and the wider society. Anthropologists have found that in many traditional communities there are beliefs that emotions pass through the milk itself. We know that breastmilk contains mothers' hormones and other substances, and also that brain scans done during breastfeeding have shown that communication centres in babies' brains become activated while close, especially in skin-to-skin, to their parents.

I found in my research with Indian mothers that they believed that feeding a child not only sustained the growth of the physical body, but also transmitted cultural knowledge about kin relations, their religion and moral values. Many mothers believe that when the baby is in the womb, he or she is experiencing the mother's emotions, and when breastfeeding, a child is learning about the world around him, through her thoughts, or in her the milk: so the future character of the child is affected by how the mother is feeling during breastfeeding.

> Most people say that if you breastfeed and you are thinking good thoughts, then he will grow up nicely, not like a hooligan who won't listen to his parents. If the mother is stubborn, the kid tends to be stubborn too. I have seen it so many times in India.[24]

In this chapter I have argued that an anthropological perspective on breastfeeding can give us insight into it being an embodied process, embedded in kinship, community and wider society. It can give us insight into it not only as an individual act, but also as binding the child to the parents, family and wider community. We can think of a body divided into the *mindful, lived body*, the *social body* and the *political body*, which could all impact on women's attitudes and experiences of breastfeeding. We need to be aware that some communities may feel that, when breastfeeding, mothers' bodies boundaries need to be protected, in order to avoid 'social pollution', and we need to be sensitive that some will not be comfortable breastfeeding in public places.

Concepts of industrial time may compel some women to restrict breastfeeding to strict intervals between feeds and length of feeds, but we could explore this with them to help them see it more as an organic, natural flow responding to babies' growing bodies.

The language, especially metaphors, we use when speaking to parents should avoid medicalising it into a mechanical process of milk transfer, but more of a close, responsive, parenting relationship. It will affect the baby's developing brain by building trust, so he becomes aware that he is not alone in the world, but his parents will respond to his needs, which is likely to have a long-term impact on his future mental health.

We need to be aware that families from more traditional societies may believe that the mother's thoughts, cultural knowledge and emotions pass to her baby through breastmilk. Perhaps, in the future, biological research may discover that this is indeed the case. Certainly, the breastfeeding hormones also have a reciprocal effect, when the mother and baby dyad are close and interacting.

You may find that some of these anthropological insights outlined can help you understand the challenges parents experience when they want to breastfeed their babies in the bottle-feeding society we currently have in the UK. Parents from different cultural groups may continue to situate breastfeeding within their organic cycle of life, which will be considered in the next chapter.

Notes

1 Bourdieu, P. (2006) *Understanding Power for Social Change*. powercube.net. IDS at Sussex University. Available at www.powercube.net/other-forms-of-power/bourdieu-and-habitus/
2 Marmot, M. (2016) *The Health Gap*. London: Bloomsbury. Available at: www.bloomsbury.com/uk/the-health-gap-9781408857991/, p. 282.
3 Bourdieu, P. (2016) *Habitus: Social Theory Rewired*. London: Routledge. Available at: http://routledgesoc.com/category/profile-tags/habitus
4 Scheper-Hughes N. and Lock, M. (1987) 'The mindful body: A prolegomenon to future medical anthropology'. *Medical Anthropology Quarterly*, 1(1), pp. 6–41.
5 Scheper-Hughes, N. (1993) *Death without Weeping: The Violence of Everyday Life in Brazil*. Reprint edition. Berkeley, CA: University of California Press.
6 Equality Act 2010. Available at: www.legislation.gov.uk/ukpga/2010/15/section/17?view=plain
7 McNish, H. (2015) *Embarrassed: Nobody Told Me*. Oxford: Blackwell.
8 Douglas, M. (1991, 1966) *Purity and Danger: An Analysis of the Concept of Pollution and Taboo*. London: Routledge.
9 Spiro, A. (2007) 'Breastfeeding in Gujarati families', in Kirkham M. (ed.) *Exploring the Dirty Side of Women's Health*. London and New York: Routledge.
10 Van Gennep, A. (1961) *The Rites of Passage*. Chicago, IL: University of Chicago Press.
11 Douglas, M. (1991, 1966) *Purity and Danger: Analysis of the Concepts of Pollution and Taboo*. London: Routledge.
12 Spiro, A. (1994) *Breastfeeding Experiences of Gujarati Women Living in Harrow*. Unpublished MSc thesis.
13 Ibid.
14 Spiro, A. M. (2005) 'Najar or Bhut – evil eye or ghost affliction: Gujarati views about illness causation', *Anthropology & Medicine*, 12(1), pp. 61–73.
15 Kahn, R. P. (1989) 'Women and time in childbirth and during lactation', in Forman, F. and Sowton, C. (eds) *Taking Our Time: Feminist Perspectives on Temporality*. Oxford: Pergamon Press.
16 Ibid.
17 Spiro, 1994.
18 Dykes, F. (2006) *Breastfeeding in Hospital: Mothers, Midwives and the Production Line*. London: Routledge & CRC Press.
19 Van Esterick, P. (1989) *Mother Power and Infant Feeding*. London: Zed Books, p. 115.
20 Tomori, C., Palmquist A. E. L. and Quinn E. A. (2018) *Breastfeeding: New Anthropological Approaches*. London: Routledge & CRC Press.

21 Maher, V. A. (1992) *The Anthropology of Breast-Feeding: Natural Law or Social Construct.* Oxford and Washington DC: BERG, p. 175.
22 Spiro, A. (2005) 'Gujarati women and infant feeding decisions', in Moran, V. H. and Dykes, F. (eds) *Maternal and Infant Nutrition and Nurture: Controversies and Challenges.* London: Quay Books, Mark Allen Publishing.
23 Spiro (1994).
24 Ibid.

11 Cultural influences on breastfeeding in the UK

The impact of culture on breastfeeding is profound, as it is influenced by deeply held beliefs which have been built up in traditional practice over generations. In this chapter, I will discuss some of the differences between white British mothers and immigrant ethnic groups, as well as those of new immigrant mothers and second and third generation ethnic minority mothers.

I will be looking at some of the research done in other countries but will focus on the main minority ethnic communities living in the UK, especially those who have their origins in India, Pakistan, Bangladesh, Africa, the Caribbean and Romania. I realise that here I can only give snapshots of some of the beliefs and practices of breastfeeding. The themes I will be looking at include: the value they give to breastmilk and colostrum; the influence of religion; the role of family members, especially grandmothers, and who makes the decision about how a baby is fed; the views about public breastfeeding; and whether views on infant feeding are changing over time. I will end with how we can, as healthcare professionals, plan sensitive support for families from different ethnic groups.

I will also draw on some of my anthropological research in North London and India; but some of my findings are unpublished, so I will just refer to the year it was carried out.

It has recently been suggested that our cultures can even change our epigenetic makeup, affecting the way our genes are expressed, which in turn, can influence the beliefs and attitudes in individual's and families' decisions about infant feeding. As healthcare professionals, we need to guard against making generalisations about a specific cultural practice or making stereotypes about an ethnic group as a whole, which could lead to us failing to understand and respect all parents' unique lived experiences. Active listening to what families are actually saying to us will help us to support them in a more appropriate way, as each one is likely to have different experiences, attitudes and practices.

What does the UK infant feeding survey tell us about the prevalence of breastfeeding in different ethnic groups?

The UK Infant Feeding Survey 2010 indicated that women from different minority, ethnic groups had the highest rates of initiating breastfeeding, with rates of over 90% in Afro-Caribbean, Chinese and Asian mothers, which is 10% higher than the national rate. The continuation rates at 6–8 weeks and 6 months were also higher in black and other minority ethnic groups.[1]

DOI: 10.4324/9781003139775-11

What does qualitative research tell us about the beliefs and practices of breastfeeding in migrant and refugee communities in different countries?

Qualitative research uses observation and interview techniques, revealing some of the beliefs, attitudes and experiences that make up their cultural milieu, which can impact on their infant feeding decisions, and family support. These insights may help us understand the attitudes and experiences of parents from different ethnicities. It may also help us plan, jointly with families, the support they may be seeking and, at the same time, not undermine their traditional practices.

An important meta-ethnographic synthesis[2] was carried out by Schmied *et al.* analysing eight qualitative and three quantitative studies from several countries, looking at the practices and beliefs of migrant and refugee women of breastfeeding, while living in their new countries. They found four main common themes: mothers' milk is best; the contradictions and conflict in breastfeeding practices; producing milk requires energy and good health; and the dominant role of female relatives.

Some of the studies they examined showed that some cultural groups carried their beliefs and practices to their new situation, but many reported a clash between these and the new dominant practices, which could lead to tensions with family members. Many of the barriers reported were similar to non-migrant women, such as returning to work, pain, perceived low milk supply and traditional beliefs and practices. They found that, despite strong beliefs in the importance of breastmilk for babies, migrant and refugee women often struggled with breastfeeding in their new host country. Some reported they had to return to paid work early and had difficulty balancing this with breastfeeding and having to fulfil household duties at the same time.

They also found some evidence which showed that as women 'acculturate' to the host country, they were more likely to take on the dominant infant feeding practices. Studies showed that, for each year a migrant mother or father resides in a new country, the duration of breastfeeding decreases. Some of the studies reported that health services and breastfeeding support were not always accessible or culturally appropriate for migrant women.

What are the beliefs and practices of migrant parents in the UK?

There are several studies of migrant parents' breastfeeding experiences, attitudes and beliefs when living in the UK, which give us some insights into how they adjust to their host countries' dominant infant feeding practices over generations. These suggest that parents and their families will differ in their attitudes and we need to guard against any generalisations and be aware of any unconscious biases we may hold.

An interesting qualitative study by Cook *et al.* was published in 2021, which investigated the beliefs and practices of different ethnic groups in the UK. It was carried out in a socially disadvantaged area of England, looking at the factors which might lead to facilitate or create barriers to breastfeeding.[3]

The methods it used involved focus groups of local mothers, after consultation with community leaders, local community groups and places of worship. They studied women whose families originally came from Bangladesh, Pakistan, Poland, some white British, and African, but found it difficult to recruit Caribbean mothers. The following is a quote from a Bangladeshi mother:

Can't do anything else around the house while breastfeeding directly, so I'm expressing so someone else can feed child. [This is] Consuming a lot of time getting him to latch on, and expressing milk takes time. It is just really difficult to manage. (Bangladeshi mother, aged 21–30)[4]

This suggested that some of the Bangladeshi women found a conflict between breast-feeding or expressing and fulfilling their household duties. The following is a quote from a Polish mother:

I believe that using formula is all the better, because it makes it all the easier for the man to help with feeding, because he can make the milk and oh, let's say that he will get up in the middle of the night and then in that instance he prevents us from getting up in the middle of the night, because he can just go on his own and do it and the child is happy and that we don't have to get up and give [food] to the child. (Polish mother, aged 21–30)[5]

Although we cannot generalise from this quote, it does suggest that some Polish mothers may be finding it more convenient to bottle feed as it gives fathers a role in feeding their babies.

As far as Caribbean mothers in the UK are concerned, repeated surveys have shown that they are more likely to breastfeed and for longer, but we do not have enough data on their beliefs, attitudes and experiences of accessing support and more research needs to be done into their lived experiences.

All the black African mothers interviewed in this study by Cook *et al.* reported that they planned to breastfeed their infants for over two years. These mothers explained that within their culture, breastfeeding was very much valued. Although breastfeeding is normal for most families in Africa, exclusivity is not common, as pre-lacteal feeds in the first three days after birth are often given and cereals may be given later in the first six months.

In many countries such as Somalia, I have heard from mothers that formula companies have been advertising artificial milk products in the last 30 years, so some women may have already been influenced by this, before they arrived in the UK.

The insights of Cook *et al.*'s study were similar to those found in the meta-analysis by Schmied *et al.* that I discussed above – that those groups who adhered to their cultural traditions held more positive perceptions towards breastfeeding; had more flexible approaches to feeding; were more likely to persevere; and many were more likely to access support from healthcare professionals. The physical barriers were similar to those found in the 2010 survey affecting many mothers in the UK. These included difficulties with attaching their babies to their breasts, with accompanying pain and concern about milk supplies; time and convenience; and embarrassment when feeding in public places.

What are the values different cultures give to breastfeeding?

The data from Schmied *et al.*'s meta-analysis[6] that we have already considered suggest that breastmilk and breastfeeding were highly valued by women from many diverse cultures, with only two studies showing that some women thought that formula milk was equivalent.

Ingram *et al.* carried out another study in Bristol[7] and found that South Asian women from Pakistan, Bangladesh and India gave cultural and religious reasons for breastfeeding. I found similar views in my research with Gujarati mothers and grandmothers living in North London and India. One mother told me that: 'Breastmilk has been given to you by the gods and you must give it to your baby.'

Ingram *et al.* also found that Somali women said they would like peer supporters from their own community who could understand their cultural preferences. A Somali mother in London told me that they have a long tradition of breastfeeding and mothers sing a lullaby to their babies while they are feeding, called 'Oh perfect child' which is 'a way of mothers praising and empowering their babies to breastfeed' (Figure 11.1).

An insightful study conducted by Burden,[8] a health visitor in Kent, included a video of the voices of Roma women, where they spoke about how they valued breastmilk and

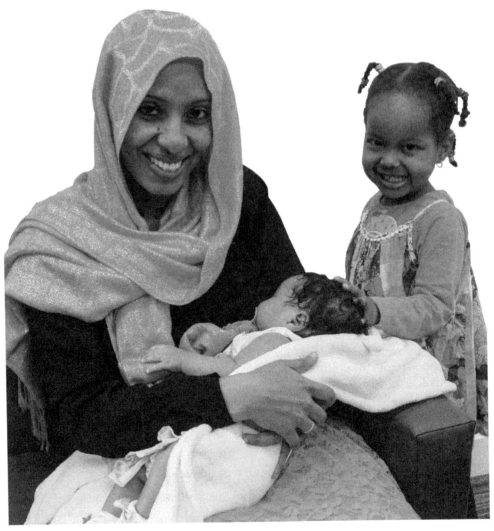

Figure 11.1 A happy family
Source: Images supplied by Real Baby Milk, a project of Pollen CIC

were knowledgeable about the benefits of it for babies. It was interesting that some had concerns about the colour of their breastmilk, which may symbolise their uncertainty of breastfeeding in the UK, where formula milk was used widely and was uniformly white. Those of you who are working with Roma families may find this video of women discussing their experiences, which are translated into English, will give you insights into their beliefs and the barriers they face breastfeeding in the UK.

Although these examples may give us a deeper understanding of women's ideas of the value of breastmilk, there may be some evidence that these may be weakening over time. We cannot assume that certain beliefs or practices are always held by individuals in any cultural groups, because every individual woman and her family will also have their own beliefs and experiences.

What is the value of colostrum?

Women from some cultural groups may be concerned about colostrum not being suitable for babies because it may contain some of the negative products from the mother's body after pregnancy and birth. We should be careful not to make assumptions about any of these beliefs but explain the value of colostrum for building the baby's immune system. The following is an anecdote of my experience of how well-meaning health professionals inadvertently created a stereotype of an assumed cultural practice:

When I started working on a postnatal ward as an infant feeding lead, I was told by midwives that Somali mothers will not give colostrum to their babies, because this was their culture which should not be questioned, so they offered them bottles of formula milk. Later, when I was training Somali peer supporters, we explored their views about colostrum and whether they would be happy to feed their babies from their breasts in the first 2–3 days after giving birth. The general feeling from the group of eight mothers was that colostrum was very important for their babies and they all said they would encourage mothers to use it.

Recently a Somali mother told me about her culture's beliefs:

They think colostrum is a good idea and very beneficial to babies, but some still believe it may not be enough. When I was a baby in Somalia, my mother breastfed me and my grandmother explained to her the importance of the first breastmilk.

I believe that ever since formula milk was advertised and mothers believing the myths of breastmilk not being enough and that babies become fat when you feed them formula. They still think 'fat' is healthy.

Interestingly, some told me later that in Somalia camel's colostrum was also highly valued and sought after for its properties of curing all diseases!

Are there religious imperatives to breastfeed?

South Asian mothers may say that there are expectations in their culture for them to breastfeed and the reasons for this may be situated within a religious context. Hindu mothers I have studied have spoken about the way breastfeeding is displayed in the iconography in temples, which they think normalises it in their culture. Some women stressed the purity of mothers' breastmilk, as a white fluid which had been given by the gods especially for their babies, so they had an obligation to give it. It had not been contaminated by being out of the body, or subjected to any processes that could make it unclean or dangerous with the gaze of jealous people, who could 'spoil the milk'.

Other mothers from South Asian countries such as Pakistan and Bangladesh have said, in Cook *et al.*'s study, that the Islamic religion was the most important influence on their decision to breastfeed. It encouraged women to breastfeed, and the Holy Qur'an states that women are expected to breastfeed for at least two years:

> Islam encourages two years for breastfeeding. Religion influences more than anything else. (Pakistani mother, aged 21–30)[9]

The close bond that breastfeeding gives between mothers and babies was seen as important from an Islamic perspective and one mother reported that:

> It makes you feel like you are serving someone else, like Allah, it is a blessing. (Bangladeshi mother, aged 31–45)[10]

What are the influences of wider family members?

A very insightful, qualitative study by McFadden *et al.* compared the perspectives of Bangladeshi women and their healthcare practitioners on breastfeeding.[11] The researchers studied 14 grandmothers who had moved to the UK in the 1950s and explored the way that living in their new country had affected their knowledge of breastfeeding. These women had left their wider kinship network in Bangladesh, which had disrupted the intergenerational transmission of the skills they needed to breastfeed. They had grown up with expectations of support with feeding their babies from the wider extended family, which were not met, leading to them feeling isolated.

The researchers interviewed 23 mothers of the second generation, who had been educated in the UK and had begun to adjust to many of the practices of this country. They told them of their needs for information and support which were often not met by healthcare professionals, as they found that the services they were offered after their babies were born were often not sensitive to their culture and family's needs.

The same study also included results from a focus group of 28 healthcare practitioners who offered care to these families, but after analysing this, it was found that they often made assumptions and used stereotypes about the women's attitudes and beliefs, rather than assess them as individuals. They made recommendations for the training of staff in cultural awareness of this ethnic group, so that service provision could be sensitive to their specific needs.

This research indicates the importance of training healthcare practitioners in the particular cultural beliefs and practices of the ethnic groups with whom they work. This could lead to them understanding what the facilitators and barriers are for these women who may wish to breastfeed their babies. This will help to plan sensitive support.

Who makes the decisions about breastfeeding?

Female relatives (mothers, mother-in-law, sisters, sister-in-law) had a significant influence particularly among South Asian, Polish and black mothers in Cook *et al.*'s, McFadden *et al.*'s and Ingram *et al.*'s studies and I also had similar findings in my research. The grandmothers, in particular, often provided important role models, following specific practices and sometimes rituals, which mothers were keen to follow. Breastfeeding was very much normalised within their families and many participants recalled experiences of watching those around them breastfeeding. This was, however, in contrast to white British Mothers where families appeared to have less influence on their decision-making. 'Mum, sister and sister-in-law didn't breastfeed, so I was nervous, they all seemed surprised that I wanted to do it' (White British mother, aged 31–45).[12]

Women from South Asia often live with their parents-in-law after marriage, leaving their own families in their country of origin and finding there could be conflicting information about breastfeeding in this country. The marriage pattern that is frequently followed is that young men living in the UK are introduced to women, or marriage is arranged with women in India or Pakistan. The wedding may then take place either here or in India or Pakistan after which the women come to live with their husbands' families, leaving their own family in their country of origin.

In one of my interviews with a Gujarati mother, I asked her who made the decisions about infant feeding and she told me:

> I don't think that Gujarati men care if their wives breastfeed or not and I think they are ignorant of the benefits. I think it is the grandmothers who pass it on and say that it is good.

Two mothers told me that they held the view that breastmilk should not go to waste:

> Sometimes when my son woke in the middle of the night, my husband would say to give a bottle, but I said no, my milk will be wasted. My breasts are full and I can't sleep.

In an interview I had with a grandmother, she said:

> You must feed your own milk because it is made specially for your child. If you breastfeed, the child knows his mother. If you bottle feed, he doesn't know his mother. If the bottle breaks, the child cries because the bottle is broken. But if the mother dies the child does not care.[13]

All the mothers I interviewed told me that it was the women in the household who decided whether to breastfeed or not. There was no conflict of the breasts as sex objects, or for feeding babies, as is the case in Western countries, but some of the older women I spoke to saw this may be changing over time in the UK. Men saw breastfeeding as residing in the woman's realm. One mother who had recently come here from rural Gujarat said:

> My mother-in-law advised me that it is best for babies' health and don't give bottles, you have enough milk. I breastfed my daughter for two years. My husband said it was up to me how long I breastfed.[14]

Somali women have told me that the women decide about how to feed their babies. The men do not usually get involved but if a woman gets divorced the Qur'an states that:

> If the wife is breastfeeding, the husband must give her due payment and treat her with kindness as always.

How can we work with grandmothers?

Those of us who have worked with grandmothers realise how important their role can be as experienced mothers, even though their personal breastfeeding experiences may have happened several decades ago. Grandmothers are often mentioned by women as the person they turn to for support, although many have not had positive experiences of breastfeeding themselves and may have found it difficult. They may want to protect their daughters or daughters-in-law from any stress and think that formula feeding may help.

If you find you have an opportunity during your antenatal visit to speak to grandmothers from all social and cultural groups about the positive benefits of breastfeeding and frequency of feeds at the beginning, it might give them a clearer understanding of the health benefits and the realities of breastfeeding babies' behaviour.

In some areas of the UK grandmothers may be more influential than others, especially when they live in extended households and traditionally play a central role in childcare. Most research in the UK has focused on grandmothers from South Asia and more needs to be done on those from other ethnic groups.

During my anthropological research with Indian families from Gujarat, in London and India, I realised how profound their influence was.

In these families, grandmothers have high status in the household. The newly married woman is cared for initially by her parents in the first 40 days after the birth of her child. After this time, she will move into her husband's home, where her mother-in-law is likely to be involved in the care of the baby. She will commonly take on roles such as bathing, massaging, comforting the baby, as well as passing on cultural knowledge by performing rituals and telling religious stories.

The father's mother often has the authority in the household to influence her daughter-in-law when feeding her grandchild. Some healthcare professionals may find this interfering and undermining the mother of the baby, but this is the expected cultural kinship hierarchy in the family.

Traditionally in South Asia there was a strong belief in breastfeeding, but after some time of living in the UK, societal attitudes and advertising of formula milk here may have weakened this and some grandmothers are beginning to think that giving babies bottles of formula may be more reliable, may fit into modern life, as well as enabling them to participate in feeding their grandchildren. Although mothers of second or third generations living in the UK will still be influenced by their mothers or mothers-in-law in this way, it may be less profound if families decide to move away from the joint household and become more independent.

This imperative to involve South Asian grandmothers in supporting mothers with breastfeeding informed an interesting study and intervention in Bristol.[15] This was carried out in an area of low exclusive breastfeeding rates. Initially, they were invited to be involved in designing a suitable programme to enable them to support their daughters or daughters-in-law with breastfeeding. Link workers from their local community were trained who could speak their languages and give them support. The health beliefs and cultural practices around infant feeding were examined by using focus groups of women from the Bangladeshi, Pakistani and Indian communities.

During the intervention, the grandmothers-to-be were initially invited to attend a focus group, when their daughters or daughters-in-law were 36 weeks pregnant, and were given a leaflet in their language explaining the advantages of breastfeeding, how babies breastfeed and what to expect in the early days. The researchers found that they were not a homogeneous group, but held different religious and cultural beliefs, which influenced their attitudes and beliefs about breastfeeding. The mothers and grand-mothers said that they appreciated the support and information they had received. This intervention appeared to be effective and influenced their attitudes and behaviour after the birth of their grandchildren, with more mothers starting to give colostrum and fewer using formula, water and dummies.

It was concluded that, for women who live in joint households, involving other family members particularly grandmothers, can increase the support women receive and improve breastfeeding rates. Effective communication with different ethnic groups may require well-informed interpreters or other community members to work with midwives and health visitors, as many of the older women may not have an adequate understanding of English.

Can breastfeeding peer supporters or doulas from different cultures make a difference?

In some parts of the UK, women from different ethnic groups are trained as breast-feeding peer supporters to work with women from similar backgrounds, which can be an effective way of giving families with new babies empathic, culturally appropriate breastfeeding support.

When I worked in the local hospital, I worked closely with a Somali peer supporter who was able to speak to pregnant women from her community in their language in the antenatal clinic and was able to give them each a copy of the Best Beginning's 'Bump to Breastfeeding' DVD (now in the Baby Buddy app) which had Somali sub-titles. After a year, audits showed that more Somali women were exclusively breast-feeding when discharged from hospital. This peer supporter was able to follow up women on the telephone if they needed extra support and visit some of them at home if they requested it.

Mars Lord, who is a doula, spoke of some of her experiences when supporting Afro-Caribbean women with breastfeeding in the UK:

> So how do we begin the conversation and education? And when do we start it? To enable us to bring breastfeeding education to future parents, supporters and advo-cates, we need to normalise it. We need to see the imagery, hear the stories and pause before either passing judgement or receiving 'perceived' judgement.
>
> What interests me greatly are the breastfeeding statistics within the black com-munity. I have spoken with people from some of the leading breastfeeding organi-sations about supporting black women and the answer always comes back, 'But they have the highest rates of initiation, so we don't think that there is an issue there'. So, the question on my mind is, 'What are the rates after initiation? At 3 months, 6 months, 1 year, 2 years, natural term?' I would love to hear your stories about your breastfeeding journey.
>
> It is easy to fall into simple rhetoric, but our words have power. People can only make informed choices when they have all the information. This means that all of the people involved in the birth of a child need to understand how and why breastfeeding works and why it is the biological norm. Cutting back support groups, healthcare professionals and resources only cripples breastfeeding rates,

and guilt, shame and/or defensiveness begin to rear their heads as misinformation is shared. So, the conversation needs to be continued. Uncomfortable truths will be spoken and many of us will have to look at how it makes us feel. We then have the responsibility of deciding how we deal with that.[16]

A study of women's experiences of breastfeeding during the COVID-19[17] pandemic showed that those from black and minority ethnic groups had more difficulty accessing support and were more likely to give up breastfeeding early. Perhaps if breastfeeding peer supporters or doulas from their own cultures had been able to give them extra telephone or online support, this might have helped them feel less isolated.

Are there cultural barriers to breastfeeding in public?

Many mothers from South Asian countries are concerned about privacy and public breastfeeding and may prefer to bottle feed in public. Some mothers decide to cover up with a shawl, or express milk, but others may be concerned about the milk becoming contaminated when outside the body. Whilst most mothers acknowledged that breast-feeding was better for the baby, formula feeding was viewed by some as a much more convenient option, especially in public places.

Some Hindu Gujarati mothers told me that even with their families they needed to be careful about where they breastfed. Some told me they were more comfortable breastfeeding in their parents', rather than their in-laws' houses.

> When I was in my mum's house, I could breastfeed downstairs and my family were comfortable about it, if I had a shawl. My dad and brothers were not embarrassed by it. My mum said that if I was watching a good film, I could stay down. But when I came home, we were sharing a house with my father-in-law and my hus-band's brother and his wife. I did not feel comfortable to feed in front of them, so I would take my daughter upstairs to feed.[18]

In my research, some Indian women told me that some believed there could be a problem of the evil eye '*najar*' if other women saw them breastfeeding in public places. If these women watching them were jealous of the way they were feeding, or the amount of milk they were making, they could cast the evil eye on them, which could spoil the milk and make either the mother or her child unwell. Many women also cover bottles of expressed milk or formula with a cloth when outside the house for this reason.[19]

Muslim women in Cook's study[20] reported that they did not find it acceptable to breastfeed in public places. My discussions with a Somali woman confirmed this:

> In the Somali community there is a stigma about breastfeeding in public. It is considered 'shameful' to advertise a modest lady breastfeeding her child.

In my experience, some other Muslim women, who wear burqas, may have slits in them for breastfeeding and can do so very discreetly without exposing any part of their breasts. They may ask, however, for a private area where they can feed, which is away from public gaze and it is important to respect this and find a private area in the clinic, where they can do this.

Afro-Caribbean women were more likely to say in Ingram's study[21] that they were confident about putting the needs of their babies above social approval, when they were away from home and their babies wanted to breastfeed in a public space.

I was told the following memories of infant feeding by a colleague who grew up in the Caribbean island of Dominica. She remembered a social difference, with wealthy families supplementing breastfeeding with formula milk. The more socially disadvantaged women breastfed their babies and there was no stigma associated with doing so in public places.

> As the eighth sibling in a family of nine, I had the opportunity of experiencing the arrival of my last sibling and sixth girl in the family, the ninth child. I was 5 at the time but have vivid memories of her arrival and the care she received following her birth. One of the things I do remember was my mother breastfeeding her initially – this did not appear to be long lived, from my recollection, as coming from such a large family and with a living-in 'nanny', my sister's care was often 'taken over' by the doting 'others' in the family – my mother must have been exhausted too – she was 45 at the time! Formula milk therefore soon took precedence over breastmilk as all her siblings literally fought to feed her, and my sister was, at a very early age, transitioned on to the bottle. During this period and later, other close friends of the family also had young babies; however, I do not recall experiencing many of them breastfeeding, and if they did it did not appear to be for prolonged periods of times. (Incidentally, my last sister breastfed all of her four children for over a year and in two cases for well over 2 years.)
>
> My experiences of breastfeeding practices in the local community particularly amidst the more socially disadvantaged groups were very different and very visible. Women sitting by the roadside either engaging in local gossip, waiting for the bus, or even selling goods in the market place very often had a young one hanging on to their breasts whilst multitasking. The ages of the young ones varied from babies to toddlers. There often was not sight of a bottle – probably because formula was not affordable, as there was a great deal of advertising going on in those days – my father being an agent for a formula company then!
>
> Later in life as a teenager, and as a young adult going back and forth to the Caribbean, my experiences continued to be varied but with more sightings of young women from my social grouping breastfeeding more 'openly'; however, babies were almost always complemented with formula milk. Nowadays, with consumerism impacting on all communities, the visibility of women breastfeeding openly in the community is not as common – I would not be able to comment on what the true incidence is – I have been told that BF is being practiced in D/CA, but with insufficient support for mothers once they are discharged from hospital – I suspect formula milk continues to reign King because of that. Whilst at home on one occasion, I was asked to see a young lady who was trying to exclusively breastfeed because she had no follow-up support.

A study of breastfeeding practices in the same island, Dominica,[22] found that breastfeeding rates were higher there than other Caribbean islands and girls were breastfed for longer than boys. In rural areas, infant formulas were too expensive, so breastfeeding was normal for the first year and there was no stigma to public breastfeeding.

Although there have been some studies done in the Caribbean and Africa, there is a lack of research into the lived experiences of these women when breastfeeding in the UK. However, there is some evidence[23] that they have problems accessing support which urgently needs to be rectified, so appropriate services can be co-created which are culturally sensitive to their needs.

Do attitudes and practices change over time and are families becoming 'acculturated'?

A study by Chowdrey found that families were influenced by the dominant feeding practices in their host countries. They looked at whether attitudes and beliefs of South Asian women change over generations while they 'acculturate' and lose some of their traditional practices. They argued that this was a more insightful way of looking at infant feeding choices, rather than just ethnicity.

This study was carried out in the UK, where 20 women were interviewed using qualitative interviewing methods to explore how their feeding intentions and behaviour changed as they became more adapted to the dominant method of infant feeding. The findings of this study showed that lower levels of 'acculturation' were more likely to draw on South Asian cultural teaching, which had a protective effect on breastfeeding.

However, women who identified more with the formula-feeding culture here were highly 'acculturated' and perceived that formula milk was more likely to meet their babies' nutritional needs and 'filled them up'. Some thought that this method was more convenient and enabled other family members to take part in feeding their babies. It also helped women fulfil their two roles of being a mother and a daughter-in-law, so they were free to continue with their household chores when they had help with feeding their babies. One South Asian mother told the researchers:

> I bottle fed my baby. It was a good experience because it was quick and easy ... my mother-in-law encouraged bottle feeding for my own benefit. I was able to share the feeding with her, which was good for me.[24]

Although this study gives us some insights into how attitudes can change over time, my research would indicate that it is a dynamic process, and many women from the same culture having different experiences and preferences. In my research, I found that Gujarati women in the UK were more likely to hold on to their traditional practices than those in India and acculturation was slow to happen. If we can focus on understanding an individual woman's and families' attitudes and beliefs, it will help us plan appropriate, sensitive support for their infant feeding choices.

How can we understand the central place of culture in women's breastfeeding experiences?

As we have discussed in previous chapters, breastfeeding in the UK has been situated here in a medical rather than a social, cultural context. Some migrant and refugee women have reported a clash between their beliefs and practices in their countries of origin and the dominant practices in their new country.

I would argue that breastfeeding has historically always been a 'cultural act', not controlled, or managed by medicine. Women have traditionally learned the 'art' from other female members of their families and communities. Mothers from different cultures speak of how they value the whole experience for mothers and babies in building relationships and transmitting their feelings, religion, family and cultural knowledge.

The focus in the UK, since the book *Breast is Best* was published in the 1970s,[25] has been on breastmilk itself, as the healthiest way to feed babies, perhaps a life-style choice, with formula milk being advertised as almost as good. There has been a failure to look at the wider social and cultural context of breastfeeding.

Although the UK UNICEF Baby Friendly Initiative has widened its focus in recent years and 'changed the conversation' with an important broadened focus on breastfeeding as important in building relationships between mothers and babies, as I have discussed in Chapter 4, here I would argue that we can extend this view outwards by looking at breastfeeding embedded in its cultural contexts. This focus would enable us to understand the impact of the deeply held practices in the UK context, with societal and political controls, on parents' lived experiences. We can learn so much by listening to parents and wider kin from different cultures about their beliefs, attitudes, cultural practices and experiences of living in multicultural Britain.

Women who come from joint families in their countries of origin, where there are close ties with kin, daily life is shared, inter-dependence is the norm, may find it difficult living in nuclear families in the UK and coping on their own with feeding and caring for their babies. They have expectations of support with caring for their infants, especially with their first babies which, if absent, can lead to feelings of isolation, postnatal depression and problems with breastfeeding.

How can we change our practice to be sensitive to different cultures?

Many of us work in culturally diverse communities, so considering some of the specific challenges faced by parents from different groups is essential for effective communication, empathic support and appropriate information sharing with them. Many black and other ethnic minority groups may find it more difficult to access breastfeeding support and many face language barriers, which can add to the inequities in health outcomes.

I hope that the qualitative research findings we have examined can suggest ways in which we can adapt our practice, by understanding how women from diverse cultures may perceive breastfeeding. We need to listen to parents' stories and enable them to identify support they might need to help them with breastfeeding. When some new parents have grown up in families where breastfeeding is the cultural norm, you will quickly realise that they are very knowledgeable about the skills and that they value breastmilk very highly.

New mothers from these groups may rely on and have expectations of family support and decisions about infant feeding, within the context of close kin networks. Working with grandmothers, as suggested in the Bristol study,[26] may help them dispel any myths they may have heard about infant feeding in the UK.

The research we discussed on Bangladeshi families[27] identified a level of apathy amongst healthcare professionals who were supporting migrant women, which was fuelled by their experiences that these mothers followed their families' traditions and disregarded professional advice. We need to understand that within this culture there may be a tradition to follow advice from family members, rather than health professionals, and interventions are more likely to be successful if grandmothers are involved in planning culturally appropriate support for their daughters or daughters-in-law.

Good relationships with practitioners were valued as important facilitators by many families in the research, which helped them to meet their infant feeding goals, by tailoring the services to support their diverse communities and acknowledging different traditional and familial practices. The recommendations of the studies were to design future programmes, which were culturally sensitive, accessible, offering materials which are translated into different languages and interpreters used when needed. Any programmes to support parents from different cultures should be targeted at reducing breastfeeding inequalities and focus on providing families with understanding, empathy, information, practical support and reassurance, not only during the early stages, but continuing through their whole breastfeeding journey.

Notes

1 NHS Digital (2012) *Infant Feeding Survey – UK, 2010.* Available at: https://digital.nhs.uk/data-and-information/publications/statistical/infant-feeding-survey/infant-feeding-survey-uk-2010
2 Schmied, V. *et al.* (2012) 'Contradictions and conflict: A meta-ethnographic study of migrant women's experiences of breastfeeding in a new country', *BMC Pregnancy and Childbirth*, 12 (1), p. 163.
3 Cook, E. J. *et al.* (2021) 'Improving support for breastfeeding mothers: A qualitative study on the experiences of breastfeeding among mothers who reside in a deprived and culturally diverse community', *International Journal for Equity in Health*, 20(92), pp. 1–14. Available at: https://equityhealthj.biomedcentral.com/track/pdf/10.1186/s12939-021-01419-0.pdf
4 Ibid.
5 Ibid.
6 Schmied, V. *et al.* (2012) 'Contradictions and conflict: A meta-ethnographic study of migrant women's experiences of breastfeeding in a new country', *BMC Pregnancy and Childbirth*, 12 (1), p.16.
7 Ingram, J. *et al.* (2008) 'Exploring barriers to exclusive breastfeeding in black and minority ethnic groups and young mothers in the UK', *Maternal & Child Nutrition*, 4, pp. 171–180.
8 Burden, P. (2019) 'Roma women talk about breastfeeding'. *CHSS Kent.* Available at: www.youtube.com/watch?v=Edn6Dy5ZLHk
9 Cook, E. J. *et al.* (2021), p. 20.
10 Ibid.
11 McFadden, A., Renfrew, M. J. and Atkin, K. (2013) 'Does cultural context make a difference to women's experiences of maternity care? A qualitative study comparing the perspectives of breast-feeding women of Bangladeshi origin and health practitioners', *Health Expectations*, 16(4), pp. e124–e135.
12 Cook *et al.* (2021).
13 Spiro, A. (1994) *Breastfeeding Experiences of Gujarati Women in Harrow.* Unpublished MSc thesis.
14 Ibid.
15 Ingram, J., Johnson, D. and Hamid, N. (2003) 'South Asian grandmothers' influence on breast feeding in Bristol', *Midwifery*, 19(4), pp. 318–327.
16 Mars Lord (2020) *Virtual Conference Baby Friendly Initiative: Doula Educator and Birth Activist.* Available at: www.unicef.org.uk/babyfriendly/speaker-series-mars-lord/
17 Brown, A. and Shenker, N. (2021) 'Experiences of breastfeeding during COVID-19: Lessons for future practical and emotional support', *Maternal & Child Nutrition*, 17(1), p. e13088.
18 Spiro (1994).
19 Ibid.
20 Cook *et al.* (2021), p. 20.
21 Ingram *et al.* (2008).
22 Quinlan, R. J., Quinlan, M. B. and Flinn, M. V. (2005) 'Local resource enhancement and sex-biased breastfeeding in a Caribbean community', *Current Anthropology*, 46(3), pp. 471–480.

23 Brown and Shenker (2021).
24 Chowdrey, K. and Wallace, L. M. (2012) '"Breast is not always best": South Asian women's experiences of infant feeding in the UK within an acculturation framework'. *Maternal & Child Nutrition*, 8(1), pp. 72–87. Available at: https://onlinelibrary.wiley.com
25 Stanway, P. and Stanway, A. (1978) *Breast is Best*. London: Macmillan.
26 Ingram et al. (2003).
27 McFadden, et al. (2013).

12 Community practitioners can normalise breastfeeding

Throughout this book I have referred to the 'time' and 'place'. A special 'time' after the birth of their baby when parents adjust to their new lives and their chosen method of feeding their babies, which I have referred to as liminal time. The 'place' where they start their feeding journey which may be in hospital, or at home, in a hostel or refuge, or even in a new country, if they are recent immigrants to the UK. Subsequently, the place where they feel comfortable feeding either at home, possibly in front of relatives, or in public areas and any cultural restraints they find there.

I have argued in this book that decisions about infant feeding are made within social and cultural contexts and if we try to understand these, by listening to families, reflecting and using empathic communication skills, we could tailor appropriate support for them. This will help us place breastfeeding back into its social context, where it is seen as a relationship embedded in culture, rather than a medical condition needing to be managed. It is so much more than a mechanical process of transferring milk from mother to baby. If new parents have not received the support they seek from families, healthcare professionals, friends or social contacts to achieve their infant feeding dreams, this could have a negative impact on their mental health and in some cases lead to perinatal depression in both mothers and fathers.

I have discussed the way that community practitioners have unique opportunities to improve the nation's physical and mental health, by supporting parents with breastfeeding, for all parents who wish to do so, by offering equity of access to support services. In the UK, we are fortunate to have the universal service of health visiting, which has as its main concern the primary prevention of ill health through the promotion of healthy behaviour and lifestyles, and offering support to all families, from all backgrounds, across the country.

Health visitors are in privileged positions to be welcomed as visitors into the homes of new families, irrespective of their social, ethnic and economic situations, so we are unique in our role of offering support with infant feeding. This service is the envy of the world, so it is essential that the government allocates sufficient resources to preserve this valued profession, to enable it to continue with this invaluable preventative service. It is vital that we all have the skills and evidence-based knowledge to offer optimum breastfeeding support to all parents, so we can work in an integrated way with other support services to enable them to build their own confidence and self-efficacy when the society and families around them may be ambivalent. At the same time, we need to be sensitive to and respect the feelings of others who are unable or choose not to breastfeed.

In this chapter, I will discuss the new government plans to support the early years through the new family hubs and the new review of the Healthy Child Programme. To

DOI: 10.4324/9781003139775-12

be most effective, community practitioners need to work in an integrated way with other breastfeeding support workers in local infant feeding teams, so parents can receive optimum support. I will explain how breastfeeding counsellors, lactation consultants and peer supporters have all received different training, and we need to understand their specific skills so we can work collaboratively with them and signpost parents to them. In this way community practitioners will find they are in positions to be able to support and assess individual families and refer them to the infant feeding team for peer or specialist support when appropriate. Through this process they can also change communities' and societal attitudes to breastfeeding.

Once breastfeeding has been reinstated as the normal method of feeding babies in the UK, it will impact on climate change by lowering carbon emissions from the dairy industry; reducing the need for the processing of formula; reducing the electrical energy used in making up feeds; and lowering the waste caused by packaging.

What are the current political policies concerning support for breastfeeding families?

In recent years, the health visiting service has been underfunded, as well as many staff redeployed during the COVID-19 crisis, which has led to shortages of staff, impacting on the support they have been able to give to parents. I have discussed how reports have shown that many new families have felt isolated and alone during the pandemic. It is hoped that the newly proposed governmental 'The Best Start' plans, with an emphasis on giving parents optimum support in the first 1,001 critical days of a child's life, will address this.[1] The new Family Hubs suggested in these plans will present opportunities for all parents to be able to access seamless, integrated breastfeeding support from their local infant feeding team, specialists and peer support.

The Institute of Health Visiting launched its 'Vision for the Future'[2] in 2019 for England, which highlighted breastfeeding as one of the 'High Impact Areas' in the Healthy Child Programme:

> Currently all parents should be offered five mandated contacts and these focus on six high impact areas where health visitors can make the greatest difference to infant, children and families' outcomes. In many areas the service is now predominantly focused on the five mandated contacts and safeguarding. However, as leaders of the Healthy Child Programme, health visitors should work in partnership with families to understand their needs and then where necessary arrange a programme of more intensive universal plus or universal partnership plus support as needed.
>
> Improving support to women to increase and sustain breastfeeding would deliver significant cost savings to the NHS and to the local authority. Reducing the incidence of just five illnesses, protected by breastfeeding, would translate into cost savings for the NHS of at least £48 million and tens of thousands fewer hospital admissions and GP consultations.[3] Premature infants who do not receive breastmilk are much more likely to suffer infections, sepsis and necrotising enterocolitis (NEC).[4]

Also, in this 'Vision for the Future', Professor Russell Viner, the former President of the Royal College of Paediatrics and Child Health (RCPCH) demonstrated his support for the service:

Health visitors act as a frontline defence against multiple child health problems – from providing advice to parents on breastfeeding and nutrition, to supporting parents with information about immunisations and safe sleeping practices. They also play a crucial role in the early identification of mental ill health, allowing those struggling to access support at the earliest opportunity. This can be life-saving. Health visitors are an important cog in the wheel that allows the child health service to effectively function. However, thanks to sharp public health spending cuts, numbers are falling dramatically, and this is having a detrimental impact on infants and children. The proportion of 6–8-week reviews completed for new-born children ranges from 90% in some areas to 10% in others for example. In its recent spending review, the Government agreed in real terms, to increase the Public Health Grant which is warmly received. In order to ensure all infants, children and their families receive the same high-level service no matter where they live in the country, the Government must reinstate the budget in full.[5]

The recent review of the Healthy Child Programme (2021),[6] emphasised the key role that health visitors have in supporting breastfeeding which is highlighted in the Early Years High Impact Area 3: Supporting Breastfeeding. This guidance explains how we can improve the health and well-being outcomes at individual, family, community and population levels.

At a family level, we play a key role in supporting parents to breastfeed and to practice responsive feeding, working seamlessly with maternity services to provide evidence-based support. We can proactively inform families where they can access peer support or specialist services when they feel they need it.

At a community level, we can 'normalise' breastfeeding by working closely with different ethnic and disadvantaged groups. We can train peer supporters from these communities, who will be able to relate to their lived experiences of breastfeeding and empathise with them. We can liaise with local businesses to offer facilities for mothers to breastfeed or express their milk when they return to work. We can work with local authorities to encourage breastfeeding in public places and provide areas in shopping centres where women can breastfeed in private places.

At a population level we can help to identify and target geographical areas where rates are lower and focus on increasing access to support there. This may require specially trained community workers or peer supporters who can make contact in settings such as homeless families' accommodation. We can ensure that UNICEF Baby Friendly training has been offered to all staff working with parents in the community, including Early Years staff, and ensure that these standards are upheld with regular training updates and opportunities for reflection and supervision.

Building an 'oxytocin society' through breastfeeding

> All of us are parents to society's children and societies must, as a matter of top priority, support parents so they can fulfil their nurturing potential. [7]

I have already mentioned Robin Grille's work about how parenting can lead to a 'peaceful world', but will refer to it again here to help our understanding of the importance of early life experiences in shaping children's brains, which then impact on their future relationships and mental health. He draws on his work as a psychotherapist in Australia and reviews recent research on the development of the human brain in childhood and the strong evidence base, on how positive, close, empathic parenting can lead to connections and 'emotional intelligence'. He argues that:

> The human brain and heart that are met primarily with empathy in the critical early years, cannot and will not grow to choose a violent or selfish life.
>
> The fact that scientists and politicians have so easily dismissed the importance of childhood as sentimentality, has enabled them to side-line some of the most critical reforms that are needed to improve children's emotional lives.[8]

Breastfeeding and skin-to-skin contact help to build relationships between parents and their babies through the closeness they bring and the secretion of oxytocin. Also, responsive bottle feeding, skin contact, carrying, co-bathing, and reciprocity can help to build closeness and empathic feelings between them. This hormone oxytocin, however, is produced in high levels, together with prolactin during breastfeeding, which helps mothers feel close to their babies.

Why is breastfeeding a human rights issue?

A joint statement by the United Nation's Special Rapporteurs on the Right to Food, Right to Health, the working group on Discrimination against Women in Law and in Practice, and the Committee on the Rights of the Child reported in 2016 on the needs for increased efforts to promote, support and protect breastfeeding.

It stated that breastfeeding is a human rights issue for both the child and the mother:

> Children have the right to life, survival and development and to the highest attainable standard of health, of which breastfeeding must be considered an integral component, as well as safe and nutritious foods. Women have the right to accurate, unbiased information needed to make an informed choice about breastfeeding. They also have the right to reproductive and maternal health services. And they have the right to adequate maternity protection in the workplace and to a friendly environment and appropriate conditions in public spaces for breastfeeding which are crucial to ensure successful breastfeeding practices.[9]

Can support for breastfeeding families become more effective through integrated working?

In the UK, we are fortunate to have many trained breastfeeding counsellors, peer supporters and specialists who can provide additional support to complement the work done by healthcare professionals. The proposed 'family hubs' that are an integral part of the early years offer by the government will provide an ideal opportunity for integrated working, so parents can access these additional services from one site.

In order to achieve these wide-ranging societal improvements, parents need to be offered consistent, integrated care pathways. There is research evidence that supports this way of working but it is important we understand each other's unique roles and training to explore the ways we could work better in teams.

An interesting study of 301 healthcare professionals attending three international conferences in Europe explored their opinions on integrated care in breastfeeding support.[10] The methodology used was asking participants to complete open-ended questionnaires which were analysed. Only the Norwegian delegates reported that breastfeeding women in their country were fully supported with breastfeeding.

The barriers they identified were that there were failing health promotion strategies, lack of vertically integrated care, and lack of shared decision-making and accessibility of information. The recommendations they drew up included that national breastfeeding committees should have roles in coordinating policies towards universal integrated support, which should follow a family-centred model. Ninety-six per cent of participants thought that integrated care was the most important aspect of breastfeeding support and 26% thought it should be incentivised within healthcare.

How can we implement integrated breastfeeding support in the UK?

Parents often complain about conflicting advice from health professionals when they ask for support with breastfeeding; integrating care with other supporters will address this. To begin with, shared local breastfeeding policies, strategies and action plans are essential. If we can join with others in training or study days, we would be able to understand each other's roles better and plan joint support offers. This quotation from the *National Maternity Review*, 'Better Births' 2016 describes the multidisciplinary approach we adopted in Harrow when I held a joint position as infant feeding lead in the community and the local hospital:

> Encouragement of breastfeeding in Harrow:
> In Harrow, a multi-ethnic London borough with high infant mortality rates, and areas of deprivation and poverty, the Director of Public Health identified breastfeeding as a top priority for 2006. A multi-professional approach was adopted with Harrow Community Health Services working with the local hospital to improve breastfeeding rates. UNICEF Baby Friendly training was commissioned for midwives, health visitors and support staff in 2007. A peer support training programme began and mothers were recruited from a local support group. A network of breastfeeding support groups was established running from children's centres, eventually achieving one every day within walking distance for all mothers. In 2008, Bump to Breastfeeding DVDs were given to every pregnant woman by midwives, health visitors and peer supporters. Harrow became accredited as Baby Friendly in 2012 and the local hospital gained the award in 2013. The staff training, peer support programme and free DVDs increased breastfeeding rates, so by 2010 initiation rates had risen to 82% and 6–8 weeks to 73%. By 2013, Harrow had 87% of mothers initiating and 75% breastfeeding at 6–8 weeks (50% exclusively), with one of the lowest drop-off rates in the UK. UNICEF assessed Harrow for its re-accreditation in 2014 and stated that it was the only local authority in the UK where breastfeeding was the 'normal' way to feed babies.[11]

How can midwives and health visitors work together more closely?

When midwives and health visitors joined together for breastfeeding training as in the above example, they found that it helped them understand each other's roles, cut down on conflicting advice and improved their communication during their handover of mothers and babies from one service to the other. In the Harrow example, the UNICEF Baby Friendly training was given in groups of midwives, maternity support workers, nursery nurses, health visitors, neonatal nurses, labour ward theatre and recovery nurses and managers. Joint strategy planning was carried out with senior hospital staff including paediatricians and UNICEF. A shared hospital and community breastfeeding policy was shared with expectant parents which quickly reduced conflicting advice from healthcare professionals, as did working together in a popular infant feeding antenatal workshop held twice a month on Saturday mornings to which parents and their families were invited. Full Baby Friendly accreditation was awarded to both trusts after eight years of this joint working.

What is this integrated approach to breastfeeding support?

It is when all workers, whether paid or volunteers, become confident about their complementary roles and can inform and refer parents for support. A case can be made to local public health departments to commission these teams. I will begin by explaining their different approaches and roles.

Breastfeeding counsellors are trained by Third Sector organisations and use counselling skills as their central approach to parents and usually work as volunteers, but some are paid to work in hospital or community settings. They are mothers who have had experiences of breastfeeding their own children, so have 'lived experience' and wish to support others. They are required to complete a course in counselling skills and practical breastfeeding skills, which usually takes two years to complete and some are university accredited.

Breastfeeding peer supporters are mothers who have happily breastfed their own children and have completed a shorter training course. The idea of turning to other women for support with breastfeeding, whether they be family members, or experienced women in the village or local community, is not new and has happened over millennia. Through the rise and popularity of formula feeding in the last century, this breastfeeding embodied knowledge has been lost to families across the world.

Most come into peer support as volunteers, wanting to enable more mothers to share their positive experiences. They complete shorter training courses than breastfeeding counsellors, commonly lasting 12–16 hours, which include the practical aspects of breastfeeding and the importance of listening to mothers, as well as the principles of counselling skills. Most of the training courses are run by Third Sector organisations such as the Breastfeeding Network (BfN), Association of Breastfeeding Mothers (ABM) and the National Childbirth Trust (NCT), who can be commissioned by local public health departments to deliver this breastfeeding peer support training, but some trusts run their own in-house courses.

Peer supporter volunteers may be still breastfeeding their own children and may wish to bring them with them to the support groups. Some are employed to work in hospitals or in community teams and will be required to complete local NHS mandatory training including safeguarding and record-keeping. Where they are working in teams, peer support co-ordinators will be essential to offer supervision and support, as well as suggested timetables. Some peer supporters may use this training and experience, even when they leave peer support, by progressing or even changing their careers to work with new parents.

Why are peer supporters so effective at supporting breastfeeding mothers?

The strength of peer supporters is that they are mothers who have lived experience of breastfeeding. They can empathise with new mothers, by putting themselves in their shoes and understanding some of the problems they may be facing. Many have had to overcome similar problems themselves and received support, but their training encourages them not to share these, but to listen to a mother's unique story. The relationships many parents have with peer supporters are ones where they feel they can speak more openly, on an equal standing, about their experiences and feelings than they can with some healthcare professionals. Thomson argued in a guest blog for the Institute of Health Visiting Voices website in 2018 that the emotional connectedness that women feel for each other when breastfeeding is very powerful and can make women feel more confident as mothers, and also more fulfilled personally.[12]

Somaiya Khan-Piachaud, a breastfeeding peer supporter, who has breastfed both of her children, told me of her moving reflections of working in this role with mothers, demonstrating what she has gained personally in this role:

> Amongst the most unexpected blessings of parenthood are the friendships that have flourished from my time volunteering as a breastfeeding peer supporter. I have met the most wonderful tribe of volunteers; and coming from a job in finance where the sector is very male dominated and transactional, it has been a tremendous privilege to work alongside some truly knowledgeable health professionals who are largely women. Approaching a new mother who is at her most vulnerable riding the post birth wave of exhilaration and exhaustion requires a set of skills beyond textbook learning. It is the soft skill of empathetic listening in a safe space of no-judgement which really gives rise to the best peer supporters.
>
> The role has helped me stop thinking about my parenting problems in an isolated way and enabled me to focus on others. The world of social media presents a very one-dimensional view of parenthood, best bits only! – and so we enter this new and unknown territory with no real roadmap or realistic expectation. Most parents-to-be are so fixated on the birth (I include myself in this) that we don't really give pause to even consider how we will feed the baby! My first son was whisked away to the hospital nursery to help me get a better night's sleep post C-section, and offered formula. It's really through the help of peer supporters that I was empowered to continue my breastfeeding journey beyond the two year mark, and my second born had the full benefit of this too with online support in Lockdown.
>
> Peer support has put me in the path of all kinds of new parents: the ones who have a thousand questions and keep coming back with more, and the ones who just need some gentle reassurance, and those who are struggling with their new identity who perhaps find the new-born haze isolating and overwhelming. To gather together and share our experiences, to see other babies of different ages and stages, and realise you are not alone is incredibly healing. Being a peer supporter continues to be my greatest honour.

In multi-ethnic communities, it is important to train peer supporters who represent their communities, understand their cultures and speak their languages. In Harrow at one stage, the peer supporter team spoke over 20 languages between them, and were able to understand some of the more complex issues the women might be facing in their family networks.

In my experience, peer supporters take their embodied knowledge into communities – even when they leave active work supporting new mothers – to their workplace, family and friends, which has a snowball effect, which spreads throughout society. Subsequently, some may even decide to pursue different careers from their previous ones, as they found that supporting new parents was so rewarding. Some may train as midwives, health visitors, lactation consultants, maternity support workers, doulas or health visitor assistants.

Do some peer supporters work as volunteers online?

There are national and international groups which focus on breastfeeding in special situations. An example of one of these is the breastfeeding twins and multiple group, which has helped many hundreds of mothers understand the extra challenges, faced with feeding more than one baby. Kathryn Stagg breastfed her own twins before she trained as a peer supporter, a breastfeeding mothers' supporter, then as a lactation consultant, and then started the national Facebook group for mothers of multiples. She has collected data to show that many begin mixed feeding their twins and triplets in hospital and after joining the group have gained enough confidence to stop the top-ups and start breastfeeding exclusively. Here she reflected on her experiences:

> Supporting twin and triplet families is so rewarding, but there are many barriers to breastfeeding multiples that may need to be climbed before it begins to become easy; 40% of twins and nearly all triplets go to the neonatal unit and the breast-feeding journey is started on the pump. Frequency and efficiency is the key in this scenario. Once the babies are well enough then the breast can be introduced gradually, but it takes a lot of time and patience for the babes to be strong enough to fully breastfeed. This can take a lot of determination and families need lots of support and realistic expectations. But with time, many of these babies can end up fully breastfeeding if that is what the parents wish.

Who are lactation consultants?

An International Board Certified Lactation Consultant (IBCLC) is usually a health professional who has specialised in the clinical management of breastfeeding and its complexity. This international training is extensive and involves hours of clinical experience with mothers. The IBCLC examiners certify those who have passed their exam and met their criteria. In the UK, some are employed by the NHS and others work privately. They are experts in practical skills, so if you have one or more in your multidisciplinary infant feeding team, you could refer mothers to them who have more complex clinical issues.

Who commissions this multidisciplinary breastfeeding support?

Public health departments have the responsibility to commission breastfeeding services as recommended by Public Health England and under the new Early Years guidance. They are required to provide evidence of the implementation of local breastfeeding policies; report on the initiation and prevalence at 6–8 weeks after birth; the duration of breastfeeding in young mothers; and those living in areas of social deprivation.

They should also ensure that the healthcare workforce has adequate breastfeeding training to support breastfeeding women, such as that provided by the UNICEF Baby Friendly initiative and support all areas to become fully accredited by them and maintain it. Lactation consultants or breastfeeding counsellors should be available for more complex situations. Infant feeding leads and support teams should be available to all mothers in your area, your managers also have obligations to follow the new NICE Postnatal Guidance (2021) and advocate for parents.

> 1.5.10 Make face-to-face breastfeeding support integral to the standard postnatal contacts for women who breastfeed. Continue this until breastfeeding is established and any problems have been addressed.[13]

How can community practitioners change societal attitudes, improve breastfeeding support for all families?

We can be catalysts for change! As the only profession that has universal contact, we are in a position to offer optimum breastfeeding support to all families. We have an obligation to ensure we all have received at least the minimal UNICEF Baby Friendly training, but we cannot all be experts! But we can refer to others who have more extensive training. We need to be careful not to undermine parents' confidence by suggesting unnecessary formula when families want to breastfeed. By working in integrated teams, we can ensure parents can access peer or expert support when needed. We can be the glue that holds the support package together for families.

Breastfeeding a child can then be realised as an achievable option for most families who wish to do it, through offering and referring to appropriate support and information. This will build their confidence and self-efficacy. Over time societal attitudes can change, as breastfeeding becomes the normal way to feed babies in the UK.

Normalising breastfeeding for older children

In some families, this may include supporting their wish to breastfeed older toddlers, or tandem feed both an older child and a new baby at the same time. Some mothers decide to continue breastfeeding while they are pregnant with their next baby and then continue to breastfeed both children (Figure 12.1). A mother told me of her experiences of tandem feeding:

> I'm tandem feeding my sons, 3-month-old baby E and 3.5-year-old Z. It was always my intention to be led by the needs of my children. I think the on-going comfort of nursing really helped Z adjust when E was born and prevent sibling rivalry. Z has never resented E or questioned why he needs 'mummy milk'.
>
> If able, Z would feed a lot more! He responds to comfort nursing and loves 'delicious mummy milk' more than anything. E doesn't comfort feed – his feeds are quick and efficient and he often just wants a 'chat' on the breast rather than gorge on milk! By contrast Z was more needy from the start and nursing solved everything. I cannot imagine mothering without breastfeeding!

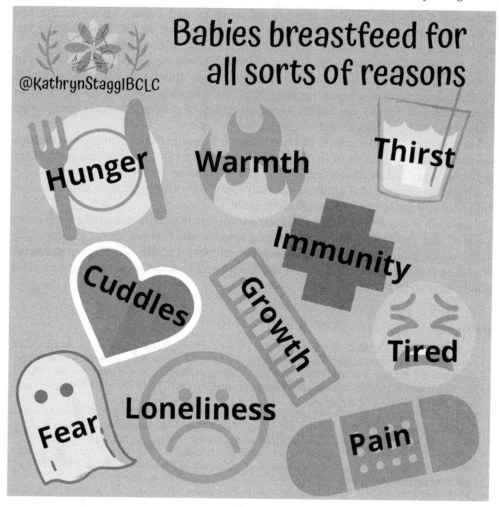

Figure 12.1 Babies breastfeed for all sorts of reasons

However, I found it much harder to tandem feed than I anticipated. My decision was not supported by most medical professionals. During my antenatal appointments I was repeatedly advised to stop breastfeeding because it might induce premature labour, but I knew this to be untrue.

I really love breastfeeding but during the last few weeks of pregnancy and the first few weeks of tandem feeding, I felt 'touched out'. This aversion soon settled and I am now so pleased I didn't wean Z until he was ready. I love how breastfeeding helps to reassure and calm my boys. It is a special gift that only I can give.

Conclusions

I have focussed on many of the health benefits as well as the wider cultural and social aspects of breastfeeding in the UK, and the way in which it can reduce social and health inequalities which have increased since the COVID-19 pandemic. The evidence surrounding how breastfeeding can protect mother's and babies' mental health has been highlighted, including its important role in promoting the lifelong health of the nation through raising mothers' and their children's physical and mental health.

As professionals working with diverse communities, we are in privileged positions of being welcomed into the homes of new families, so our attitudes and listening skills will be crucially important when supporting them with feeding their babies. We need to understand and respect the beliefs and experiences of different cultural groups and address any implicit bias or stereotypes we might hold.

There are many wider effects of breastfeeding: it protects the environment, through reducing carbon emissions in the processing of formula milk; the plastic waste needed in bottles, teats and sterilising equipment; and reliance on the dairy industry.

It upholds parents' and children's human rights by enabling parents to reach their infant feeding goals, through optimum support.

Above all, it is a loving way for parents to care for their babies, meeting their needs for food and comfort while building strong attachments between them, so promoting their infants' brain development and future good mental health. When parents cannot or choose not to breastfeed, they can still build these close relationships through close skin-to-skin contact and responsive feeding.

Notes

1 Gov.UK (2021) *The Best Start for Life: A Vision for the 1,001 Critical Days.* Available at: www.gov.uk/government/publications/the-best-start-for-life-a-vision-for-the-1001-critical-days
2 Institute of Health Visiting (2019) *Health Visiting in England: A Vision for the Future.* Available at: https://ihv.org.uk/wp-content/uploads/2019/11/7.11.19-Health-Visiting-in-England-Vision-FINAL-VERSION.pdf
3 Renfrew, M. et al. (2012) 'Preventing disease and saving resources: The potential contribution of increasing breastfeeding rates in the UK', UNICEF, p. 104. Available at: www.unicef.org.uk/wp-content/uploads/sites/2/2012/11/Preventing_disease_saving_resources.pdf
4 Colaizy, T. T. *et al.* (2016) 'Impact of optimized breastfeeding on the costs of necrotizing enterocolitis in extremely low birthweight infants', *The Journal of Pediatrics,* 175, pp. 100–105.
5 Institute of Health Visiting (2019).
6 NHS England (2021) *NHS Healthy Child Programme.* Available at: www.healthychildprogramme.com/
7 Grille, R. (2005, 2008) *Parenting for a Peaceful World.* The Children's Project. Available at: www.goodreads.com/work/best_book/1762776-parenting-for-a-peaceful-world
8 Ibid.
9 Office of the UN High Commissioner for Human Rights (OHCHR) (2016) *Joint statement by the UN Special Rapporteurs on the Right to Food, Right to Health, the Working Group on Discrimination against Women in Law and in Practice, and the Committee on the Rights of the Child in Support of Increased Efforts to Promote, Support and Protect Breast-feeding.* Available at: www.ohchr.org/en/NewsEvents/Pages/DisplayNews.aspx?NewsID=20871
10 Rosin, S. I. and Zakarija-Grković, I. (2016) 'Towards integrated care in breastfeeding support: A cross-sectional survey of practitioners' perspectives', *International Breastfeeding Journal,* 11(1), p. 15.
11 NHS England (2016) *National Maternity Review Report.* Available at: www.england.nhs.uk/wp-content/uploads/2016/02/national-maternity-review-report.pdf
12 Institute of Health Visiting (2018) *Breastfeeding Peer Support.* Available at: https://ihv.org.uk/news-and-views/voices/breastfeeding-peer-support/
13 National Institute for Health and Care Excellence (NICE) (2021) *Recommendations: Postnatal Care. Guidance.* Available at: www.nice.org.uk/guidance/ng194/chapter/Recommendations#postnatal-care-of-the-baby

13 Breastfeeding support organisations

The Association of Breastfeeding Mothers (ABM) (charity): abm.me.uk
Helpline: 0300 330 5453, plus its counsellors also work on the National Breastfeeding Helpline.
Some local support groups.
Leaflets for sale.

The Breastfeeding Network (BfN) (charity): www.breastfeedingnetwork.org.uk
Runs the National Breastfeeding Helpline: 0300 100 0212.
Drugs in Breastmilk service.
Provides extensive information, including drugs factsheets, and expressing and storing breastmilk information on its website and as leaflets.

La Leche League GB (LLL) (part of LLL International) (charity): www.laleche.org.uk
Helpline: 0845 120 2918; some local support groups.
Extensive range of books and sheets for sale.

National Childbirth Trust (NCT) (charity):
The UK's largest charity for parents, incorporating skilled breastfeeding support in a range of services, such as antenatal courses and introduction to solids workshops. www.nct.org.uk
Helpline: 0300 330 0770; provides support in all areas of pregnancy, birth and early parenthood, including feeding.
Extensive information on website.
Baby Café is part of the NCT group: www.thebabycafe.org

Lactation Consultants of Great Britain (LCGB): the professional organisation for UK IBCLCs (International Board Certified Lactation Consultants). www.lcgb.org
Search facility for IBCLCs on the website.

Association of Tongue-tie Practitioners (ATP)www.tongue-tie.org.uk
Search facility for tongue-tie practitioners on the website.

UK breastfeeding helplines

National Breastfeeding Helpline 9.30am – 9.30pm	0300 100 0212
La Leche League GB (LLLGB)	0345 120 2918
La Leche League Northern Ireland	028 95 818118

DOI: 10.4324/9781003139775-13

NCT Helpline 8am – 12 midnight	0300 330 0700
Breastfeeding Helpline for Bengali/Sylheti speakers	0300 456 2421
Breastfeeding Helpline for Tamil/Telugu/Hindi speakers	0300 330 5469

Breastfeeding Network (BfN): Drugs in Breastmilk Information www.breastfeedingnetwork.org.uk/detailed-information/drugs-in-breastmilk/drug-information@breastfeedingnetwork.org.uk

Index

Entries in *italics* refer to figures.